YOGA AND THE ART OF
MUDRAS

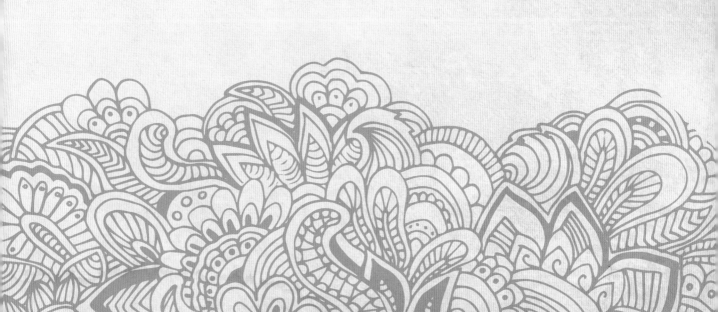

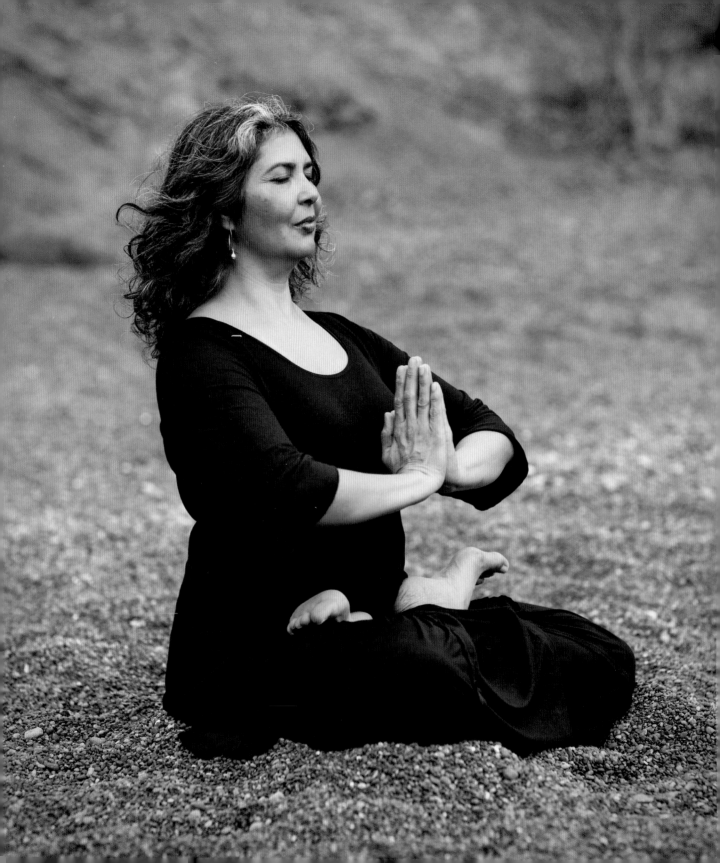

YOGA AND THE ART OF
MUDRAS

NUBIA TEIXEIRA

PHOTOGRAPHY BY ANDREA BOSTON

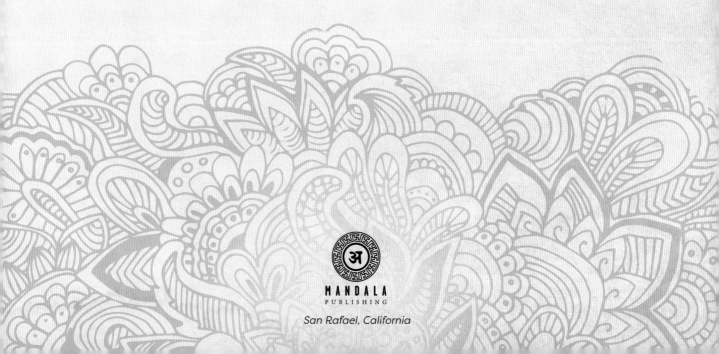

MANDALA
PUBLISHING

San Rafael, California

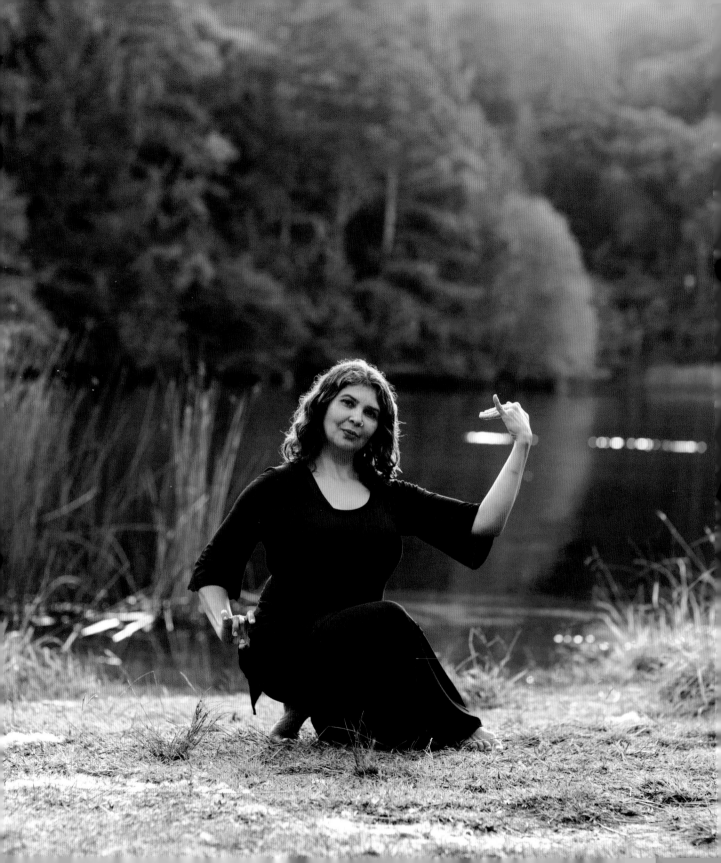

CONTENTS

PREFACE

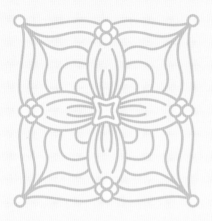

From a very young age, I have been drawn to work with my hands and intrigued by the power of this vehicle of my own body. I grew up in São Paulo, Brazil, and as a young woman looking for a way to deal with my emotions, I ventured into the realm of theater. Through voice projection, hand gestures, and body movement, theater practice taught me a way to redirect my misunderstood feelings into something positive and meaningful by acting them out. It showed me how my passions and my fears intertwined and sprang from the same source within me.

At the age of sixteen, I started practicing hatha yoga, which brought nourishment to my body, mind, and heart. The tradition provided me with a new language that was supportive of my deeper spiritual pursuits. Through my yoga practice, I was able to tap into the "soul within the body" and found a path to the sacred and the devotional within. The practice of yoga made me curious about my inner life and the world of mysticism. I devoted hours of my day to the practice and study of yoga and its philosophy and became interested in investigating a more subtle realm by deepening my yoga practice.

I studied yoga for four years at the Universidade de Yoga, in São Paulo. There, I was educated in the Swasthya yoga system, which is divided into eight main practices: mudra (hand gestures); puja (acts of worship); mantra (sacred sound); *pranayama* (breathwork); *kriya* (cleansing techniques); asana (postures); *yoganidra* (guided visualizations); and dhyana (meditation). During those four years, I learned how to link body, energy, and spirit and discovered the link between yoga and art. Since that time, my yoga teaching style has always tended to include mudras as part of the opening ritual, and I also always add mudra to mantra and *yogasana* practices.

Yoga had become my healing art and my dharma, and I knew that I had found a new way of expressing the artist within me. Yoga helped me feel balanced and strong in my body and gave me the ability to perceive and channel spiritual and healing energies sourced from the ancient well of this practice. I received benevolence and support from my teachers and felt the responsibility to share this gift with others. Since the beginning, my goal with yoga has been to support my students in aligning their physical bodies with their hearts and supporting them on their spiritual paths. I have also always wanted my students to experience beauty and to feel loved. When adjusting my students in yoga poses, I always made sure that my hands are filled with loving healing energy, as I consider it to be my service, or *seva*. Therefore, my mastery of Reiki only came to reinforce this call I felt to serve, work, and heal with my hands.

When I traveled to India, I was exposed to various classical Indian dance forms. Being exposed to the Odissi dance of Eastern India in particular, I was fascinated to see the devotional mood with which the dancers would tell stories, translate their prayers, and invoke the gods and goddesses, all by using their hands. To me, the language of the hands was much more captivating than all the hard work the dancers were doing with their bodies and feet. The dancers' hand gestures were breathtaking and hypnotic, and the magic of their shapes and movements transported my eyes and spirit to a parallel mythical universe. It was one of the strongest impressions I can ever remember having in my life, and I felt I had found my pot of gold. So much richness filled my days, and the path of Bhakti Yoga entered my life through the medium of devotional dance.

My experience with dance deepened my relationship to the power of the mudras in my life and guided me to use the hand gestures not only as expressive art and a means of prayer to the Divine, but also as a way to help my students infuse and embellish their yoga practices with all of these influences. Through my daily spiritual practice in the form of prayer, dance, and yoga, I increasingly began feeling the presence and blessings of the divine gods and goddesses in my life, and as a result, I felt ready to introduce some of my sadhana as a devotional component to my yoga classes.

After an enriching trip to India, during which time I was able to fully absorb myself in the practice of yoga and the study of dance, I moved to California to be with my husband, Jai Uttal. Along with the gift of uniting with the love of my life, Jai, I was brought to Neem Karoli Baba's feet. I had the honor to witness Jai's daily devotion to his guru and to learn about the practice of Bhakti from Jai's perspective, experience, and complete devotion. I saw that Maharajji's all-embracing presence was orchestrating all the events occurring in our lives; I immersed myself in Maharajji's Bhakti, and by his blessings, Jai and I were gifted with our beautiful boy, Ezra Gopal. Motherhood is for me the highest form of yoga. Being a mother, being Ezra's mother, has taught me so much and allowed me to experience a type of unconditional love that I had never felt before.

Over the years, I have continuously studied both yoga and dance under the tutelage of traditional teachers. I have also immersed myself in the art of Reiki and Tantric Buddhist healing methodologies, and in so doing, I have devoted myself to creating a system of healing arts that is rooted in tradition but incorporates influences from various different cultural sources. It is my objective to offer a personal and authentic practice of what I call embodied Bhakti Yoga.

This book is an expression of all of these various influences in my life. Within these pages, I offer some of the most beautiful gems from my collection of mudras and asanas—a collection that has been inspired by over twenty-five years of experiences, practice, and teaching. Most of the hand gestures are combined with yogasanas and inspired by Odissi dance postures. My sincere dedication and deep love for the two paths of yoga and Odissi have brought this humble offering into being, and my prayer is that within these pages you will find inspiration to infuse your practice with devotion, magic, and art.

Any mistakes I've made will hopefully fall at the feet of the One I serve.

With love and respect,
Nubia

INTRODUCTION

An Offering from My Heart to Yours

"yatho hastato dhrishtihi
yatho dhrishtisto manaha
yatho manatato bhavaha
yatho bhavastato rasaha"

"Where the hands go, the eyes will follow
Where the eyes go, the mind will follow
Where the mind goes, the emotions are awakened
Where the emotions are awakened, rasa arises."

—*From the* Natya Shastra, Abhinayadarpanam

This book is a simple offering introducing my vision of integrating yogasana with mudra and Odissi dance shapes. My aim is for this book to serve as a resource for yoga practitioners and yoga teachers alike and show a way to teach them how to grace their yogasanas with mudras that come from a traditional source. As a yoga teacher and trainer of teachers myself, I know there's a need and a desire for this kind of material. As a *yogini* who believes in preserving the deeper traditions and yet also feels comfortable blending schools of thoughts, I want to inspire and empower others by showing what is possible when yoga, mudra, and Indian dance come together.

These mudras are not mine; they belong to the tradition of expressive art and classical Indian dance sourced from the *Natya Shastra* of Sage Bharata Muni and the work of *Abhinayadarpanam* of Nandikesvara. Mudras have been taught as a way to express and tell stories that increase morality, awaken the heart, and orient both the performer and the audience toward union with the Divine. The first chapter of the *Natya Shastra* beautifully explains the origin of the power of words, stories, and movement, which I share with you here, in my own words:

Once upon a time, Indra, the god of the heavens, and other devas approached Brahma, the god of creation, with a request: "We desire to have our stories retold. It is our wish that these inspirational tales become popular and that people of all castes have access to them." Brahma looked at the gods in front of him and replied, "So, it shall be." Seated in his yoga posture, Brahma summoned, in his mind, the four Vedas and then said, "Let me create the fifth Veda; it shall be called Natya (drama), and, combined with the stories of the epics and sacred scriptures, this Natya Veda shall awaken virtue by art, wealth by practice, and spiritual freedom by grace." The benevolent Brahma then created the Natya Veda by drawing forth the words from the Rig Veda, the singing from the Sama Veda, the hand gestures from the Yajur Veda, and the flavors from the Atharva Veda. And, having done so, the Brahma said, "May this body of art be the source of counseling for all flavors (rasas) and all moods (bhavas) and be expressive of all actions (kriyas). It should serve as a resting place to all in need, grieving, weary, or unhappy. This book will reunite everything that is separate, bestowing union (yoga) to lover and beloved. I made this book for all seven lands, for the mortals and immortals, and in accordance with the world's order (svabhava). May the weals and woes of humanity be expressed in art through the movements of the body, in worship (puja), and in total devotion and surrender."

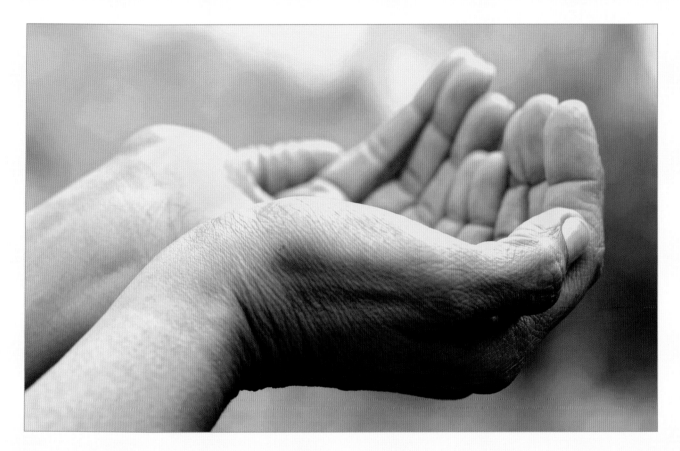

Bringing these symbolic mudras to yogasana is somewhat new, although it has been done before. Still, the compilation in this book is very personal to me, as I used my own artistic discretion to match each mudra with each pose. Before making my statements in this book, I made sure these compositions were strong and filled with meaning, allowing the practitioner to use their body in their heart's offerings.

In this book, I also present a new repertoire of yogasanas as based on the Odissi poses of some of the main gods and goddesses of the Hindu pantheon. These asanas are expressions of these deities and the embod-iment of their instruments, symbolism, and properties. I call them *bijasanas*, or "seed poses," and they contain the latent potency of these divine beings. Each bijasana either represents an aspect of a deity's power or tells a story from an episode of the deity's life. Practiced with devotion, these special poses become a way to tap into the well of generosity of these divine beings.

In the Indian dance tradition, we learn long and complex pieces, which are sacred, filled with meaning, and most often follow a Sanskrit prayer (sloka). These pieces, which can last anywhere from five to twenty minutes, contain elements of pure dance (nritta) and expressive story lines (nritya). Inspired by the shapes and moods contained in these sacred dances, I plucked a few of the most beautiful flowers, and they became the bijasanas found within these pages.

The Body

The purpose of our yoga sadhana is to awaken awareness of many parts of ourselves and endeavor to unite them all. Within the philosophy of yoga, the practitioner is encouraged to perceive herself as having five layers of being: physical, energetic, mental, causal, and eternal. For the purpose of this embodied Bhakti Yoga practice, we will first concentrate on three different parts of the body to start with the attempt at uniting them.

We often take for granted the privilege of having a functioning physical body and forget that this precious incarnation of ours is sacred. If you reflect for a moment on all the factors that were involved in finding the right time and place for you to be born, the perfect and the imperfect conditions of your family, and the qualities of character that would support your evolution as a spirit in this body, you would probably give more credit to your body and honor your functioning physical body as a sacred gift.

We often go about our day, doing what we do, unaware of this extraordinary companion to our soul, namely the physical body. Workaholics ignore the body because the task ahead is more important than the needs of this unique companion. Others pay attention to the physical body only when they feel pleasure or pain. Still others focus only on the physical attributes of the body, obsessed with maintaining its youthfulness and, at the same time, fearing its demise. Many more will identify themselves with the external—what they can see, feel, and immediately experience, and forget that they are made of many more layers—that the body houses the spirit and the soul, and that it is accompanied by an emotional heart and a wise mind.

Some spiritualists ignore the body entirely, believing that they are not the body and implying that the body is somehow less honorable than the spirit. In saying the body doesn't matter, they have forgotten what is speaking. It is the body that speaks, and it relies on an entire network of interdependent organs and instruments to do so. From the muscles to the mind, from the lungs to the voice, the body comprises a whole, allowing one to speak.

This work is an invitation to infuse this human body with sacred beauty and geometry—a practical guide with inspirational "seats" to support our bodies as instruments for certain qualities, energies, emotions, and virtues you may wish to develop and nurture.

The Hands

The hands, which are an extension of the heart center, can carry the energies and prayers of our innermost sanctum outward and, in turn, bring into our hearts the energies and prayers that sustain us. Our hands connect us to the outer world; they are the instruments we have for how we reach out, touch, express, heal,

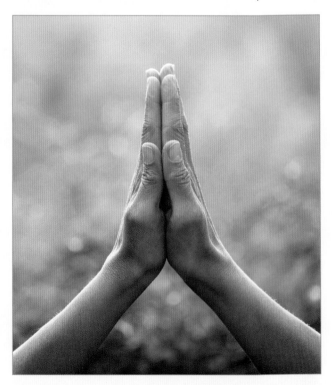

work, cultivate, cook, paint, write, play music, and hold one another. Our hands often reveal our innermost thoughts and feelings; they can convey ideas or opinions, show directions and instruct others, and allow us to communicate with one another. Our hands can bring abundance to our lives through the work we do and by the way we express our hearts. Reflecting on this fact helps us appreciate just how much of what we do in this world is enabled by our hands.

Like the power within the words we speak, our hands possess the power to manifest our thoughts and actions, positively directing them to bring virtue and beauty into our lives and into the world around us.

With our hands, we can access the unseen and reach for spiritual support and orientation. With our hands, we can touch and help one another, empowered by the ever-present love within our hearts. We choose that love to seed our actions, and we choose to be of service as we spread this love out into the world. Manifesting our reality within each action we take, we hope that everything we touch will turn into gold love.

The Eyes

The final and most important part of this work is to awaken the power within the eyes and their potential to reveal our innermost feelings and self. Mastering the eyes' expressions in the practice of dance is the most advanced part of dance, and this is comparable to the practice of concentration, also known as the *drishtis*, within the hatha yoga tradition. The eyes reveal the soul of the person, their deepest intention, and an ancient longing for union.

Yoga Sadhana

Sadhana means your daily spiritual practice; it is the method you use to understand your true nature. One's yoga sadhana provides the means to discover the union between the individual soul and the eternal soul—in other words, to discover yoga.

There are many different practices nowadays that come under the umbrella of yoga, so a yogic sadhana repertoire can be diverse, complex, even divergent, and that's OK.

Understanding our individuality in relation to humanity can become the starting point of our yogic journey. As we identify our own real needs, our deep-rooted tendencies, and our psychophysiological makeup, and as we discover our physical bodies, our wounds, our gifts, and so on, we can choose the practices of yoga that will support us to evolve as spirits within this body.

There is never only one aspect of truth or one way of practicing yoga. Rather, there are many roads and many ways of practicing that lead toward the one and only universal truth. What we learn through our sadhana practice of self-study will hopefully ripple outward and help us see the diversity of creation without judgment and embrace the differences between us and others as elements that complement rather than divide.

The goal of our spiritual daily practice, our sadhana, is to come to a place of ease within ourselves and with the world around us. We can practice yoga by doing one more positive action and one fewer negative action every day. That will help us become increasingly aware of the purity of our own hearts and of the qualities we wish to embody and express. Some of those qualities include being receptive and able to set boundaries; being loving and protective, kind and truthful, and peaceful and strong; and serving humanity as we take refuge in and surrender to the Divine.

I support you in creating your own mission, and I encourage you to offer that mission as the seed of your intention during your yoga sadhana.

Bhakti Yoga

"Bhakti Yoga awakens the devotional heart and kindles the quality of love inside of one's inner being, resulting in external acts of love and service."

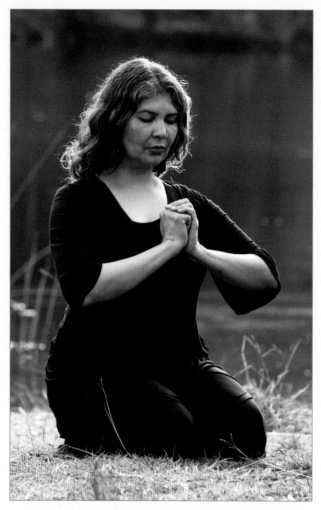

into our hearts and to honor our feelings and emotions by channeling them as fuel for our devotion. I personally chose Bhakti Yoga to be the foundation of my practice and my teachings as it allows the yogini or yogi to offer to the Divine whatever one can offer in a number of loving ways.

My own Bhakti comes from my personal relationship and experience with the sacred, from the heart awakenings I have felt through my solitary conversations with the mother goddess, and from having met so many inspiring Bhakti yogis and saints who have changed my life and awakened the devotional love in my heart in a very special way.

Saints, poets, and yoginis of the past have inspired and guided so many toward the blessed realm of Bhakti. By their own devotion, personal experience, and accumulated dedication, they have obtained the grace of reunion; by their generosity, they grant us access to their merits so that we may come to realize and benefit from a small fraction of their wisdom. This is called grace.

We can bring Bhakti into *all* of our relationships: with the Divine, with ourselves, with one another, and with Mother Nature's entire creation. We can express Bhakti in everything we do—from waking up in gratitude to sleeping as an offering, from awakening in *seva* (selfless service) to reuniting in faith and total surrender. Acting in this way is a simple and direct way of tapping into an ancient well of benevolence, light, and remembrance. Bhakti reminds us that each relationship with the Divine is unique and can only be expressed by the individual bhakta. In order to do this, however, you must fully embrace all that you are, create conditions that align yourself with the Divine, and offer your thoughts, words, and deeds into that light of wisdom and love.

Intertwined with Bhakti Yoga is karma yoga, or the yoga of "selfless service to God," through service to humanity and to the planet. This path is critical in these times and an important way to support life and to care for all living creatures on this planet. The essential meaning of karma yoga is to act in devo-

Bhakti Yoga is an ancient path of yoga, considered to be the most effective in this era of Kali, or darkness, because it can guide those who practice it toward the great salvation of divine love. *Bhakti*, often translated as "devotion," is a type of practice that allows a practitioner to develop a personal relationship with the object of devotion, the deity being worshipped, or both. For many other paths of yoga, attachment is perceived as an impediment to enlightenment. Within the Bhakti Yoga tradition, however, faithful attachment to the object of devotion can lead a bhakta to union with his or her chosen deity. Bhakti Yoga invites us to bring light

tional service and without expectation of reward. Neem Karoli Baba said to his followers, "Feed people and love them," or, "Love everybody, serve everybody, and remember God." I take that lesson as my main orientation on karma yoga.

Infuse every act, including your yogasana, with the sincerity of your heart. With that authentic love flowing from your devotional heart, go about your day doing whatever you can do to benefit others. As Krishna says, in the Bhagavad Gita, "Better to fail doing what you must than succeed in a dharma not your own, for that way is dangerous" (Joshua M. Greene, *Gita Wisdom* [San Rafael, CA: Mandala Publishing, 2009], page 18).

Ultimately, experiencing the Divine in our day-to-day life, in everything we do, and in everyone we see is part of the goal of reuniting, or yoga. This goal can keep us on track and inspire us to be the best we can be at all times. Slowly and skillfully, we can create the conditions that lead us toward this objective.

Asanas in Yoga

"Evolution is the fruit of a sincere and dedicated practice."

Hatha yoga was originally taught by Shiva, or Adinath, the first yogi and the first dancer. Shiva's dance of the tandava is associated with dissolution, and the original intention of yoga was to bring about transformation, freedom, and reunion with God.

One legend says that while Lord Shiva was teaching the secrets of yoga to his beloved consort Parvati by the shores of the ocean, a tiny fish was peeking out of the water and listening to Shiva's instructions. Every day, the fish would receive the teachings and immediately swim back down to the bottom of the ocean to faithfully practice what he had heard. This little fish, or Matsya, became the lord of the fish, a perfected being known as Matsyendranath.

Originally, the practices of hatha yoga were designed to prepare the committed practitioner to reach the more advanced states of consciousness and move into higher levels of awareness. In the *Hatha*

Yoga Pradipika, we find a list of fifteen yogasanas suggested by Swatmarama, plucked out of the eighty-four yogasanas that Shiva taught to Parvati. These fifteen asanas combine yogasanas with the yoga mudras of the body, which are also called *karana mudras*.

Transporting the practices of hatha yoga to the current age, it's logical for us—as a culture and society in which women and householders practice hatha yoga—to set more realistic goals for our hatha yoga sadhana. These goals, infused with a more feminine, intuitive understanding of the practice, would include bringing both strength and flexibility to the body and mind; refining balance, establishing stability, and cultivating harmony; being receptive to divine inspiration, orientation, and reconnection; and finally being open to love—open to selflessly serving others and supporting them in their lives. Think of asana as a medium for the study of the self or soul, or a seat from which to evoke balance and peace. Multiple asanas can become remedies, too, as different parts of the body are activated and different effects can be experienced within each unique posture.

I feel that yoga and yogasana are universal blessings. I perceive asana to be timeless, boundless, independent, interdependent, and practical. Witnessing Mother Nature express herself in her totality, diversity, and complexity teaches me how to be more embracing of the infinite possibilities. Creation is bountiful, and the variety of shapes and species that we can find in nature remind us of how many asanas are fashioned in the fullness of her myriad expressions.

Having been birthed from the womb of Mother India, yoga has grown beyond its Indian boundaries to bless all of humanity. It is important for each one of us to respect the origins, traditions, and the original spiritual intention of the ancient yoga practice while also honoring our own cultural background, ancestry, body types, and special needs. With all that in mind, we can then apply ourselves to practicing yogasana in our unique way and with our own chosen sadhana.

The yogasanas give us a place from which to start our inner work, and then from the physical body we can access all the other layers of our existence. Beginning with the focal point in your physical body, you can shift the awareness to your body of energy and into the feelings, emotions, and sensations stored in your *pranic* body.

From the body of energy, you begin to witness the waves of thoughts and the recollections of the body of mind and choose to look into the space between those waves. Moving into the layer of the body of wisdom and higher mind, you can come into contact with your intuition and have the opportunity to transmute and evolve as a spiritual being. This may allow you to develop the ability to receive the grace to glimpse into the layer of bliss within.

Strong and flexible in your asana, move through this world with presence, awareness, compassion, philanthropy, availability, understanding, acceptance, and appreciation.

Mudras in Yoga

"Therefore the goddess sleeping at the entrance of Brahma's door should be constantly aroused with all effort, by performing mudra thoroughly."

—Hatha Yoga Pradipika (3.5)

Mudras, literally imprints, stamps, seals, or hand gestures, are a powerful set of physical tools that can be used to influence and activate the flow of *pranic* energy within the yogi's subtle body, mind, and psyche. These hand gestures can function like electrical plugs, granting access to the energy of whatever you want to connect with. For example, by assuming Shiva's mudra and meditating on it, you will be plugging into Shiva's domain and accessing information from his spiritual legacy. In the Tantric tradition, from which hatha yoga derives, mudras combine with the chanting of a mantra and the visualization of a yantra during sacred and secret rituals.

In the Gheranda Samhita 3:4–5, Lord Shiva describes the meaning of *mudra* to Parvati:

"mudranam patalam devi kathitam tava sannidhau yena vijnatamatrena sarva siddhih prajayate gopaniya prayatnena na deyam yasyakasyacit pritdam yoginam caiva durlabhamarutamapi"

"O Devi! I have imparted the knowledge of mudras. Mere knowledge of these provides siddhis, mastery. Their knowledge provides bliss to yogis. Their knowledge is not easily accessible even to gods. Keep this knowledge always secret."

—Gheranda Samhita

Although in hatha yoga mudras are of two types—*hasta mudras*, or hand gestures, and *kaya mudras*, or postural mudras—in this book, we will focus only on the yogic hand gestures and on how these hand gestures work as keys to unlocking inner states of awareness, turning on spiritual abilities, and awakening some specific qualities within our psyches.

Focusing on the hands as an extension of the *anahata* chakra (the heart), where the element of air is more present, we can enter the realm of interconnection with all forms of life and connect to the flow of life force. In the center of the chest, we witness a constant dance of contraction and expansion, revealing the pulsation of life and the power of movement. Depending on its quantity and the quality, the prana that circulates in the chest supports and inspires transformation and allows us to connect with the realm of the spirit.

In the physical body, the element of air (*vayu*) is felt by the skin (organ of perception or *jnanendriya*), activated by the hands (organ of action or *karmendriya*), and sensed by touch (*sparsha*). The yogini will feel the well of life force in her heart's vortex, and she will focus on developing the qualities of the heart and on expanding her extrasensory abilities.

Air links the invisible to the visible and carries the forces of the mystical reality into our material world. The sense of touch can be felt physically, energetically, mentally, and spiritually. Within our hands and hearts is a vast sky, and the connection to the heavenly realms and celestial beings can be established through mudra.

Mudras in the practice of Bhakti Yoga become offerings from your individual soul to the universal soul. When you hold a mudra of a specific deity, you don't become that deity but your action allows you to come closer to their domain. The key hand gestures become a conduit for their auspiciousness to flow to you, so you can feel their presence within you. The mudras grant you access to experience the grandiosity of these gods and goddesses—in small doses—and, by way of transmission, to become their instrument.

Intentional mudras can be used to balance out the extremes of your personality or your disposition. For example, if you know that you have a big ego and tend to be self-centered, be careful not to feed that quality; when performing a bijasana (pose of the deity) don't assume that you are the chosen god yourself. Instead, as you come closer to the deity's domain, approach

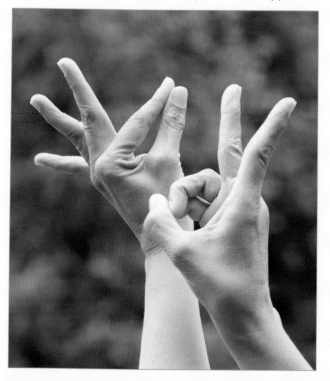

with humility, ideally as a servant. On the other hand, if you have a tendency to be shy or have low self-esteem, you can use the mudras to emulate the great power of the divine—to evoke the presence of a great goddess within you so she can empower you physically, allowing you to feel her force and echo her voice. With this personal experience imprinted in your heart, you can then be empowered to be your strong true self.

Each mudra in Bhakti can be a key into a mythical gate. It can bring a bhakta onto the doorsteps of a divine being's abode, and it can support a practitioner to channel the essence of their chosen deity (ishta devatta). Holding the key can allow you inside of the temple, but please remember to be a respectful guest in that sacred space. Remember, it is an honor to come that close to the inner sanctum, and it is a blessing to be able to feel a small fraction of the power of the Absolute for even a fraction of time.

I urge you to apply to your practice of the mudras to faith, humility, and devotion.

The *Hastas* of the Dance Tradition

Many of the mudras in this book are part of the vocabulary of hand gestures that compose the language of abhinaya or *hastabhinaya*—storytelling using the hands. *Abhi* means "toward," and *ni* means "to carry." Abhinaya is a theatrical and artful expression that is intended to convey to the spectator the sentiment (*bhava*) and flavor (*rasa*) of the message and the mood that the artist is feeling and channeling.

Each *hasta*, or hand gesture, may reveal a symbol, creature, element of nature, myth, mood, deity, or something else. The *hasta* connects us to that which is being evoked by the hands, and it is an offering to the sacred—a means of reverence, or a way to channel and express all of the divine plays. *Hasta mudras* are ways of praying, praising, and communicating with the Divine and with life. One of the things I love about them is that they support me in my offerings without the need of doing anything external. For example, if

I would like to offer a garland of flowers, I can do so without ever having to pick or buy flowers. Using my imagination and my hands, I pluck flowers from a tree, thread them into a garland and, in my mind's eye, offer them to my chosen deity.

Abhinaya is a language in itself, and the rudiments of this form of expression started long ago with Lord Shiva performing his dance of tandava and with Goddess Parvati responding to her beloved's dance with lasya. The tandava is the divine dance of Shiva, and it is a vigorous, ardent, and blissful dance. The lasya dance is filled with beauty and grace, and it reveals Devi Parvati's sensual mood and aesthetic toward her lover, Lord Shiva. The combination of yogasana and *hasta mudra* in this book is deeply influenced by this dance tradition, which can be traced back to lord of the dance and master of yoga himself, Lord Shiva.

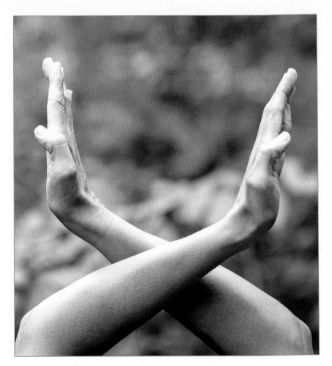

> *"padatalahata patita shailam*
> *ksobhita bhuta samagra samudram*
> *tandavanrttamidam pralayante*
> *patu jagat sukhadayi harasaya"*

> *"May the tandava dance of Shiva, as it crushed*
> *the mountains with the stamping of his feet,*
> *agitated all beings and all the oceans (by the*
> *swept movements of his hands) and protect*
> *the world after the deluge and bestowing*
> *happiness on it."*

—Rangacharya, 2011

Hand Gestures of the Abhinayadarpanam

The *Abhinayadarpanam*, literally "the mirror of gestures," by Nandikesvara, is a compendium taken from the scripture of the *Natya Shastra* of Sage Bharata. It describes in detail the art of dramatic science, which uses the movements of the body and many other elements of the expressive arts. I relied on the authority of this scripture to bring forth the bijasanas, the seed poses or seat poses of the deities. Almost all of the bijasanas formulated for this book, with a few exceptions, follow the prescription of the *Abhinayadarpanam*'s manuscript.

In the abbreviated treatise of *Abhinayadarpanam*, we find enough material for a lifetime of work. We will learn how to articulate almost all of the diverse human and divine moods (*bhavas*) and many of the extensive variety of feelings and flavors (*rasas*). The text introduces particular rites, crafts, gods and goddesses, and human beings, as well as the kaleidoscopic spectrum of nature, including the many animals and other forms. It teaches us how to express the many actions of humans and how to enact the different phases of one's life.

With the support of the *Abhinayadarpanam*, an artist can be capable of embodying a poem, prayer, or sacred text and bringing to life the essence, the meaning, and the teachings of that which is being staged.

The hand gestures are closely tied to the Hindu iconography found in so much of Indian art and in the sculptures of the Hindu deities. In both art and Bhakti, the hand gesture is associated with the blessing being given; in other words, it's a way to link the appreciator to the energy of whatever or whoever is being appreciated. What is revealed to each bhakta may be different, but the essence and meaning of the mudra is always the same.

When performing these hand gestures or watching someone perform them, keep the mirror of your heart clear, and open your inner eyes to see beyond the form into the essence of what is being evoked. Allow yourself to penetrate, via these seals, the sanctuary of your soul and, from that place, access mystic reality. You might receive darshan, or a divine appearance, in return.

The Classical Indian Dance of Odissi

> "Jagannath svami nayana-patha-gami
> bhavatu me"

> "May Sri Jagannath, the lord of the universe,
> be the object of my vision."

Odissi Dance is a highly sculpturesque classical dance form from the state of Odisha, an eastern Indian state on the Bay of Bengal. Although the intention of this book is not to teach you Odissi, I would like to introduce it because many of the poses and mudras that we use in this book come from this source.

Odissi in its essence is devotional. Like most other Indian classical arts, this dance was born inside the temples and has a deeply spiritual component. Many temples exist in Odisha, but the main ones are the Jagannath Temple in Puri, the Lingaraja Temple in Bhubaneswar, and the Konark Sun Temple in Konark. Archeologists have traced Odissi back to the caves and temples; by the time this art form was carved in the columns of the temples, it was already a fully developed dance system.

In the temples of Odisha, especially in the Sun Temple in Konark from the fourteenth century, inside of the hall of dance or *natya mandapa*, one can see hundreds of sculptural reliefs of women holding different dance positions and hand gestures. The vocabulary of the hand gestures and movements of this dance method is exquisite and graceful, and to be able to see these shapes engraved inside the temples is a timeless gift for lovers of the sacred arts.

Lord Jagannath, the spiritual patron of Odissi dance, is an expression of Sri Krishna's form known as Mahabhava-prakasha, or the manifestation of the highest mood of ecstatic love. In the temple of Jagannath in Puri, the temple dancers, called *maharis* or *devadasis*, performed Odissi. These "servants of God" lived in devotion to their Lord Jagannath and enacted their ritualistic dance-prayer exclusively within the inner sanctum as part of the temple's daily worship. They performed only to delight Lord Jagannath, mostly before his bedtime.

We dancers today benefit from the *maharis*, who lived their lives in worship to the Divine through the dance of Odissi. The *maharis*, after a marriage-like ceremony of commitment to a lifetime of service to Sri Jagannath, became initiated in the arts of music, dance, and ritual. Their offerings were an essential part of the daily temple worship, and they held a place of prestige in society. This sets the tone and the purpose of the classical dance of Odissi: dedication to one path, commitment to the sacred arts, and devotional service.

Throughout it's history, Odissi as a living art has had many different influences, including the intimate stories of the Gita Govinda, the ecstatic Vaishnava dharma of the saint Chaitanya Mahaprabhu, the invasion of the Moguls along with British colonization, and many more. During this period, as the devadasis were taken out of the temples and not allowed to perform their sacred rites anymore, young dancing boys, or *gotipuas*, were trained in this art. They preserved the tradition and also influenced it with more of an acrobatic style.

The guru of all my gurus in Odissi, Kelucharan Mohapatra, was a *gotipua* himself. He dedicated his entire life to this sacred art. Sri Kelucharan, along with other renowned Odissi dancers, formed an association and worked together to further refine this art form.

Subsequently, in 1957, Odissi was recognized as one of the main classical Indian dances.

My Odissi dance teacher, Sri Vishnu Tattva Das, explains, "Today, though Odissi dance has stepped out of the temple into mainstream society, it continues to inspire and awaken beauty and grace in the hearts of artists and spectators alike. In increasing numbers it is brought to life through dedication and devoted work, allowing it to evolve and thrive as it passes from teacher to student, building a future with ancient history and culture into the new millennium."

Odissi in My Life

I was exposed to the many different Indian dance styles in my first trip to India in 1997. I was studying yoga during the day and going to music and dance performances at night. When I returned home, I was determined to find a teacher to train with. I found Sonia Galvão. While watching her performance, I fell totally in love with Odissi, ran backstage, and inquired about learning from her. Sonia became such an inspiration to me, giving me so much structure, content, correction, and information. She taught me by example the importance of discipline and devotion to an art form.

I went deep and devoted many hours of my day for many years to building the shape of Odissi in my body. Then, when I went back to India, where I lived for six months and danced Odissi every day, dance became a gateway into the world of symbols and mythic reality. I noticed its transformational power in my life, from simply feeling better in my body and clearer in my heart to finding a spiritual shelter and a deep well of inner abundance. The treasures that were manifesting in my awareness were not of this world, and yet they enriched my inner and outer lives so much, with supernatural and invisible support.

The dance is built in your body from your feet up to your head. Like the construction of a temple, the foundation is the most important part to establish, then the walls of the temple can be erected, and eventually all of the ornamentation will be placed upon a strong structure. I remember in the beginning how hard it was for me to move in the way I was being asked. The hands had to go one way, while the legs had to move in the opposite direction. The gaze had to follow the hands, and the feet had to follow the beat. I had to sit in a deep, ballet-like

plié, and I could not move my hips, which was difficult for a Brazilian who grew up dancing samba. I had to develop calluses in my feet in order to stomp on the ground, and I had to be OK with aching muscles as I held my arms up and kept my knees bent—seemingly forever. And yet, I was in bliss. All these initial challenges just strengthened my respect and love for this devotional expression and intensified my desire to learn more about it.

Later on, studying Odissi with Sri Vishnu Tattva Das has brought so much depth to my practice, and the classical Odissi repertoire is finally rooted in my body and heart. Odissi in my life is pure inspiration, a home-coming to an artistry that felt ingrained in my bones. I invite you to see through this art form the beauty of nonlinear expression and the divine perfection of a golden ratio of proportions. Look for the details of the shapes as they reveal the meaning of the sacred geometry of the yantras and mandalas and grant you access to the supernatural realms and the abode of the deities.

How to Use This Book

"If one offers me with love and devotion a leaf, a flower, a fruit, or water, I will accept it. Whatever you do, whatever you eat, whatever you offer or give away, and whatever austerities you perform—do that as an offering to Me."

—Bhagavad Gita 9.26-27

This book opens with ritualistic yoga: poses and mudras practiced as a way to worship the five elements—earth, water, fire, air, and space. Working with these poses will give you an idea of how to perform your daily puja and how to begin your daily yoga practice. You can choose to work with one element at a time or all of them within a single practice.

Next comes a sequence of meditative yoga: poses and mudras combined to give you different qualities to reflect upon. To figure out which one to work with, spend some time contemplating which properties you need the most, and begin with the seats that support balancing your predispositions, helping to enrich your inner life.

Finally, a tapestry of yogasanas and bijasanas are woven into the sequences to create what we may also call *mudrasanas*. Mudrasanas are a combination of hand gesture and poses, and these combinations are put together to reveal a story. Bijasanas are the seed power pose of each deity. Like a seed contains the power of the tree, these poses contain the power or the quality of the deity being evoked. In this section, you will notice that specific yogasanas are grouped with relevant bijasanas since they relate to the deities' stories.

The yogasanas I chose are simple and always include a variation suitable for beginners so that they are appropriate for all students new to asana.

I'm not as interested in describing the *anatomical* alignment of each pose as I am in encouraging you to find the *spiritual* alignment. Even though the more advanced hatha yogis may want to explore different, perhaps more advanced, expressions of the pose, they must always remember to prioritize the aspect of devotional art and the embodiment of the *rasas*. I hope that these formulas can help you draw inspiration from the intangible and connect you to nature's miraculous source.

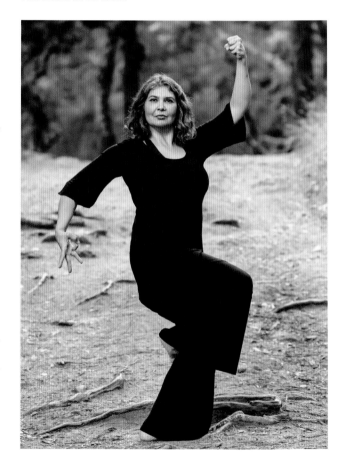

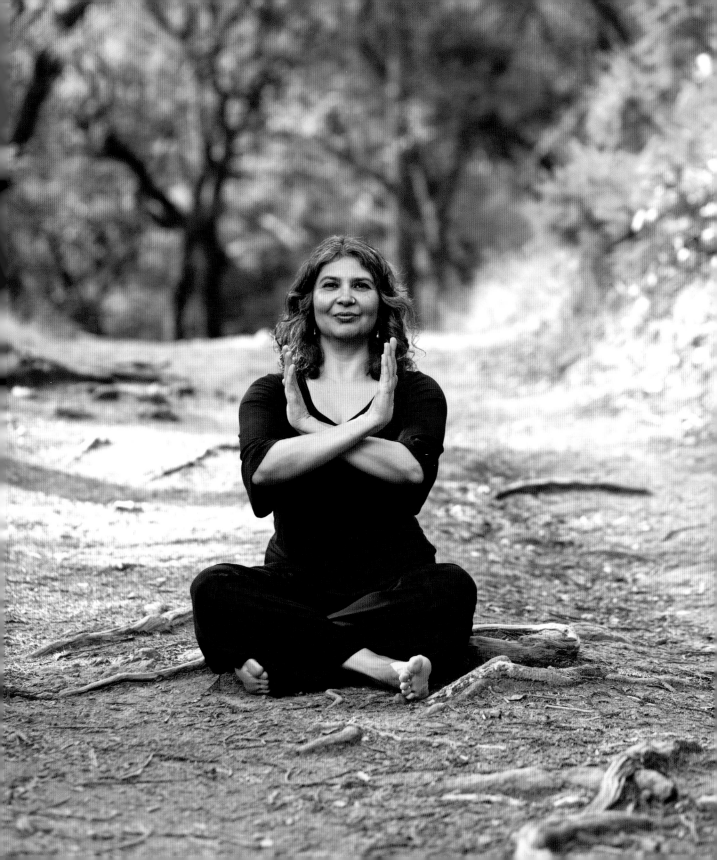

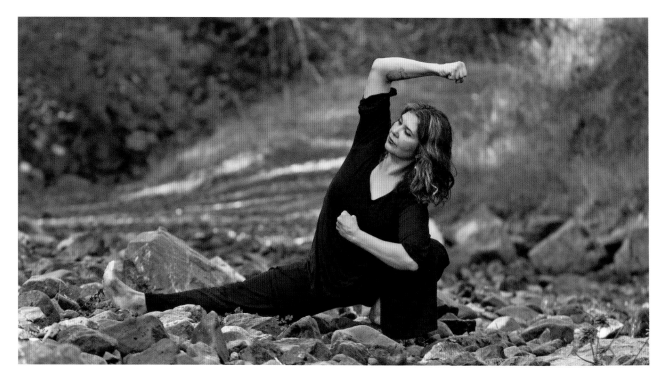

For the bijasanas, many of the asanas are based on the different *padas*, or foot positions, and *pithas*, or seats of the Odissi tradition. I carefully chose one physical asana that would encompass a distinct deity's main property, and I used the mudras prescribed by the *Abhinayadarpanam* for that deity.

I've grouped the poses according to which deities need to be categorized together as families. For example, Parvati stays with Shiva, Vishnu with Lakshmi, Sita with Rama, Radha with Krishna, and so on.

Each one of the poses will act as host for the visitors you are consciously summoning with your hands. Practice these poses by withdrawing your senses and bringing your attention to the world of symbols; this will enable you to access the collective unconscious and unveil sacred mysteries and inner truths.

You will begin by focusing on the physical body, and then, as you firmly anchor in your form, you can add the mudra, feeling the key-like power of that hand gesture to open the gateway to your devotional heart. After

that, as you hold the pose with the mudra, you evoke in prayer the qualities you wish to cultivate within your body, mind, and heart. From your foundation—the physical earthliness of the body—open layer by layer to the cosmic expansiveness of your soul.

You will, in time, begin to perceive these asanas as pieces of sacred art and practice these shapes to call upon and channel primeval energies that will enrich your life and your yoga sadhana.

I humbly hope that you will cherish these gems that I have collected, reshaped, polished, and shared with you, and that they will give you a little taste of my big love for these practices.

As you begin your journey through this book, first look at all of the photos of the poses, from beginning to end, so you can assimilate this visual and poetic guided journey by awakening the senses, igniting your imagination, and sparking your inspiration.

After looking throughout this book as a visual experience, I would like for you to start by reading the meaning of the mudras on each page. Take the time to practice each mudra and to meditate and create a relationship with each one of the seals individually.

If you are new to yoga, I would like for you to please take the time to practice each one of these poses individually and, if necessary, seek the guidance of a local yoga teacher to help you to polish your asana shape. I have added a brief description of the asanas, and if you need more details or have any concerns and or special needs, you should look for a yoga professional to support you with that.

If you are already a yoga practitioner and know the yoga asana poses, you can go ahead into the next step of combining yogasana and mudra. After becoming familiar with mudras and asanas separately, bring them together in your practice, and feel the alchemy of these two conduits operating as one, namely mudrasana.

Then begin by learning the compositions gradually, only moving on to the next when you fully embody the prior, using these vessels for contemplation and channeling. Focus on deepening your relationship with each one of these configurations, slowly becoming attuned to the essence of what you are evoking through the body.

For all the poses, remember to compensate: Do the same pose or hand gesture on both sides of the body. Although it is not scripturally traditional to perform some of the bijasanas on both sides, I suggest you do it for the sake of the body's balance. With some bijasanas, I offer a different mudra for the other side, so pay attention to that. For example, in the *Shiva bijasana*, Shiva will be holding different mudras on each side.

Each pose has a theme and intentionally calls upon a specific sentiment or deity, stimulating the heart of the practitioner and opening the worshipper to the many possibilities of revering, communing with, and creating devotional art. Allow your body to experience the mood and feeling of each pose, and call upon the energies I've suggested while allowing room for your own personal experience and inner truth.

My hope is that this collection of mudras and asanas will inspire you on your yoga path, supporting you in finding new ways to connect to the sacred through the body. As you express your devotional art and deepen your personal relationship with the Divine, may you find happiness and success.

I hope that sharing the art of the hand gestures may benefit the yoga community and, in turn, extend outwardly toward many other art forms. I pray that our practice will connect us to the natural forces of creation, sustenance, and dissolution and that the rituals presented here will empower us to unveil the mystical world for our own salvation.

I pray that the divine beings summoned here will support us as we navigate this human incarnation. May they guide us toward transcending our limited understanding of who we really are so that we can prioritize our spiritual and inner lives while we are situated in this material existence.

I pray that throughout this life we can find a way of mirroring through our speech and actions the purity and beauty of our tender hearts and unleash from within the transformational force of unconditional love, now and forever.

"Spread the seeds of devotion upon this beautiful earth of ours."

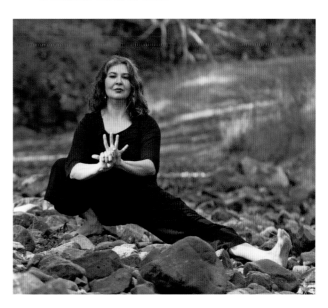

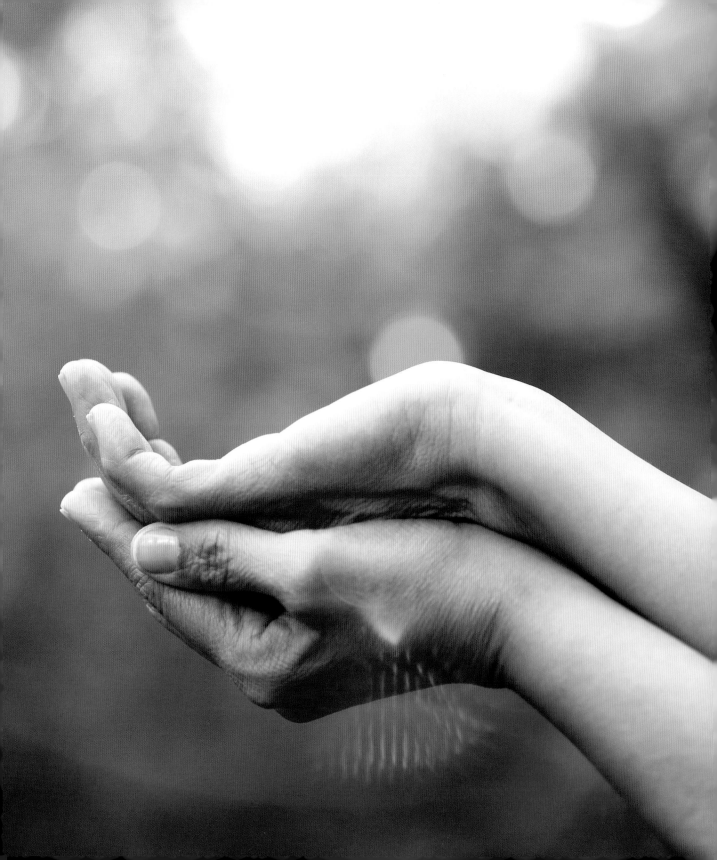

Opening Prayer
Asking for Blessings

· ·

To start this journey, I am asking for the blessing and mercy of our spiritual guides, saints, and divine beings:

May we, through our bodies, develop the qualities of poise and strength.

May we, through our words, express the qualities of truth and kindness.

May we realize within our heart the qualities of wisdom and love.

May we work together to bring beauty and inspiration to our lives and to the lives of those around us.

May we follow the orders we receive from our teachers and act on our spiritual and mundane duties.

May we find joy and peace within our hearts and bring more goodness and light to this world.

RITUALISTIC YOGA

Honoring the five elements

In this opening section of our yogasana practice, we will honor the five compositional elements by dedicating simple offerings to them. Everything in this manifest world is composed of a mixture of the five elements: earth, water, fire, air, and ether, the latter of which is the subtlest. Ritual offerings are called *pujas*, and they are to be done with a sincere heart and an internal attitude of devotion. The offered items are visualized and prepared internally and presented externally with our hands and through our actions.

These simple rituals, inspired by the Vedic tradition, can be part of the opening practice of your yoga sadhana, or practice, but they can also work as independent invocations for purification. Aim to hold each of these poses for a period of one to two minutes each.

From gross to subtle, we find a way toward emancipation and reunion, and from subtle to gross we find a way toward manifestation and cocreation.

To the earth, I offer sandal paste, or gandha.
To the water element, I offer food, or naivedya.
To the fire element, I offer light, or deepa.
To the air element, I offer incense, or dhupa.
To the ether element, I offer a flower, or poola.

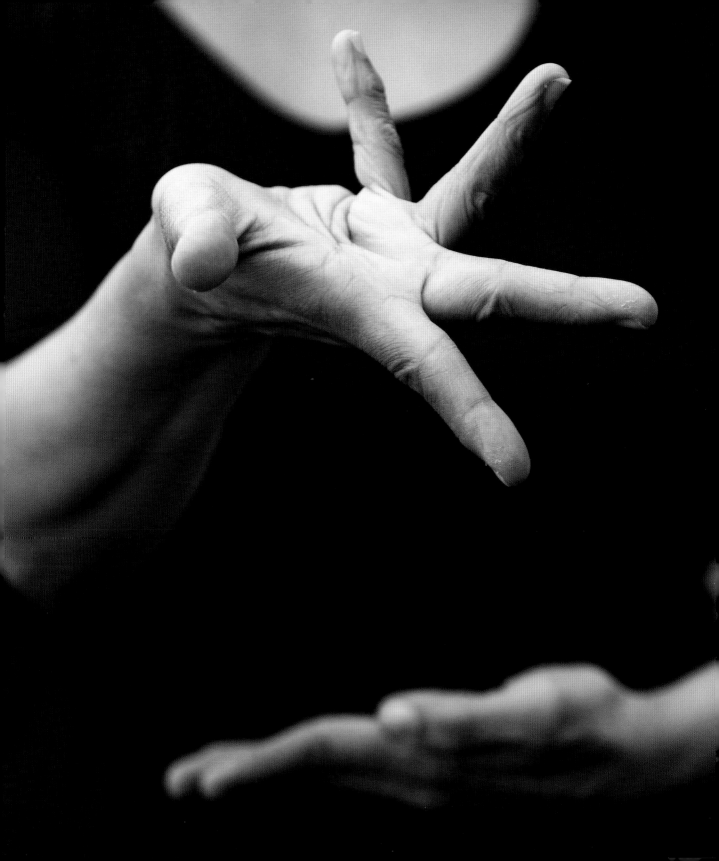

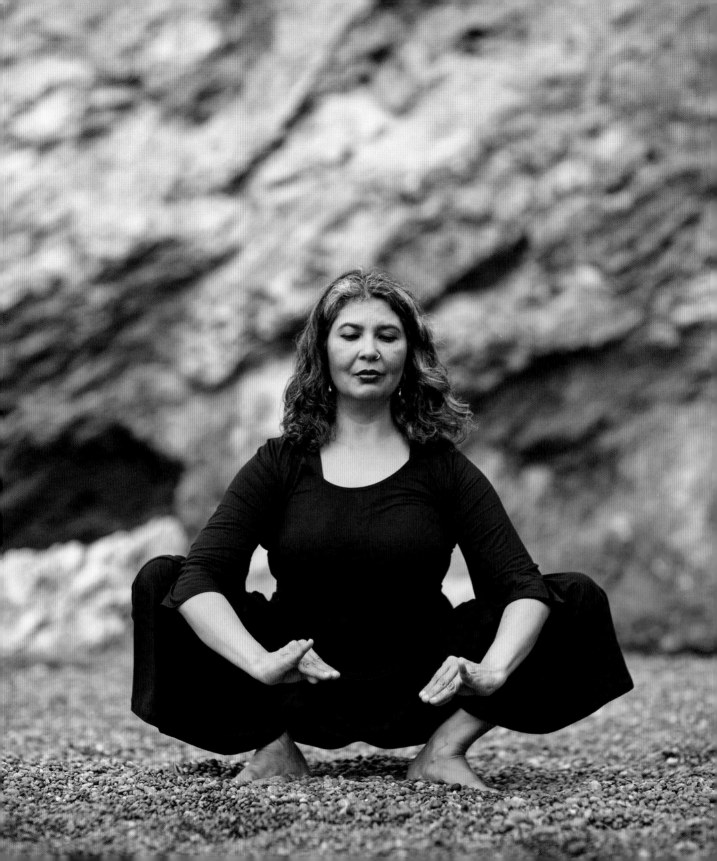

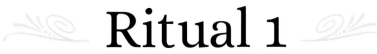

Ritual 1
Prithvi, the earth element
Malasana with *chatura mudra*

Mudra

Chatura symbolizes a square, and it is a formal way of touching the earth as part of the earth salutation, or *Bhumi pranam*. Place your thumbs at the base of the ring finger, and lift your little finger high and straight up to the sky while stretching index, middle, and ring fingers forward.

Asana

From standing pose, separate your feet to align with your hips, and turn your feet and knees slightly out. Squat down, and keep your spine straight. If needed, support your heels with a folded blanket. You may also like to place a folded blanket behind the knees.

Ritual

Salutations to the earth element and salutations to she whose body is the earth:

> *"With gratitude in my heart to have this body and to be on this earthly plane, I take refuge on your earthly lap, oh Mother, and I ask you to please take over my ego and guide me."*

To the earth, I offer sandal paste, or *gandha*.

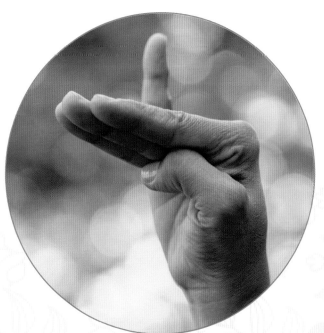

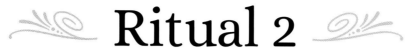

Ritual 2
Apas, the water element
Ardha kumbha pada with *pushpaputa mudra*

Mudra

Pushpaputa symbolizes the act of offering, and in this case we are offering water with our imagination. Through our small offering, we connect to the abundant waters within our physical body and with all bodies of waters above and below the earth. Keep your fingers together, and make the shape of an offering bowl with your hands.

Asana

From standing pose, feet one wrist's width apart, turn your feet and knees out and as you bend the knees to sit on your heels. Elevate the heels and open up the knees while keeping the torso upright. For variation, after sitting in *kumbha pada*, you may lower one of the knees to the earth and flow from one knee down to the other down, like a watery dance.

Ritual

Salutations to the water element and salutations to she whose body is water:

> *"With gratitude in my heart to be able to feel your qualities moving through me and to carry your waters, I take refuge on your watery lap, oh Mother, and ask you to please grant me the power of discrimination between right and wrong."*

To the water element, I offer food, or *naivedya*.

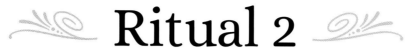

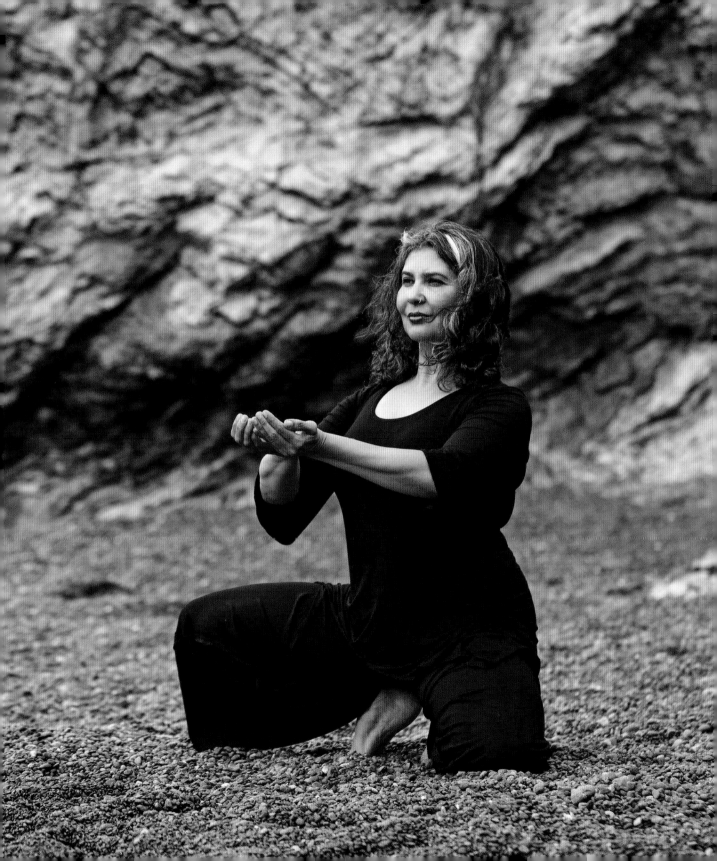

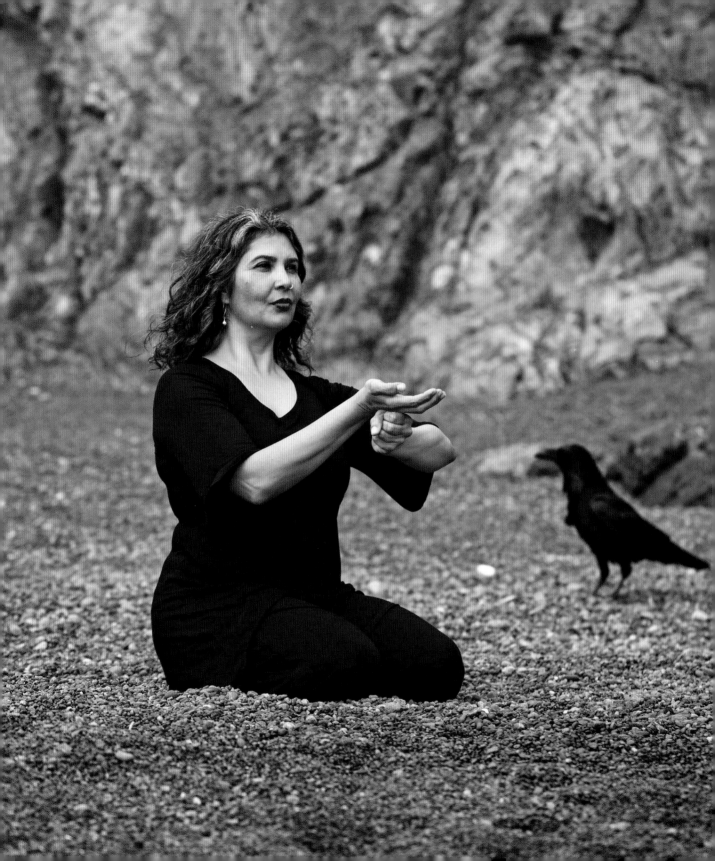

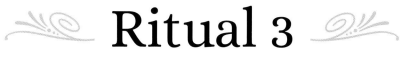

Ritual 3
Agni, the fire element
Vajrasana with *pradeepa mudra*

Mudra

Pradeepa means "lamp" or "light," and in this ritual, you are offering light unto the element of fire. With one hand, make a fist, which is the base of your lamp. With the other hand, make a shallow bowl, which is the top of your lamp. Visualize the light in your hands as you make this offering.

Asana

Sit on your heels, keep your feet together, and place the tops of your feet on the ground in thunderbolt pose. If needed, prop your hips by sitting on a folded blanket or block. Keep your spine upright and belly relaxed.

Ritual

Salutations to the fire element and salutations to she who is the power of fire:

> *"With gratitude in my heart to be activated by your heat, I take refuge on your warm lap, oh Mother, and I ask you to please be the object of my focus and purify my mind's heart."*

To the fire element, I offer light, or *deepa*.

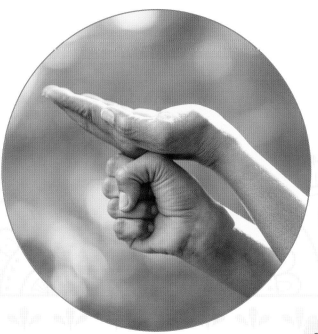

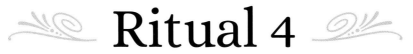

Ritual 4
Vayu, the air element
Vayutkatasana with *kapittha mudra*

Mudra

Kapittha in this ritual is the mudra symbolic of the holding of incense. With one hand, point your thumb up and place the tip of your index finger on top of it. During your *puja*, you can wave your hand, as if you are waving the incense in the air.

Asana

This is the pose of the power of the wind. Stand with your feet slightly apart, and bend the knees while sitting on your heels. Maintain a balance, and keep your knees pointing forward, such that the heel supports the sitting bones. This pose requires the practice of maintaining balance.

Ritual

Salutations to the air element and salutations to she who is the breath of air:

> *"With gratitude in my heart for the ability to feel the spirit and the life force moving through me, I take refuge on your airy lap, oh Mother, and I ask you to please bless me with the wisdom of your love."*

To the air element, I offer incense, or *dhupa*.

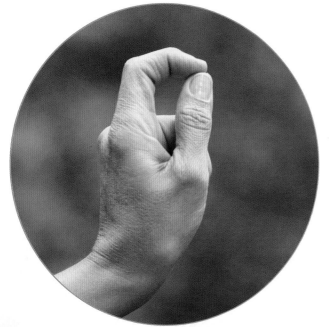

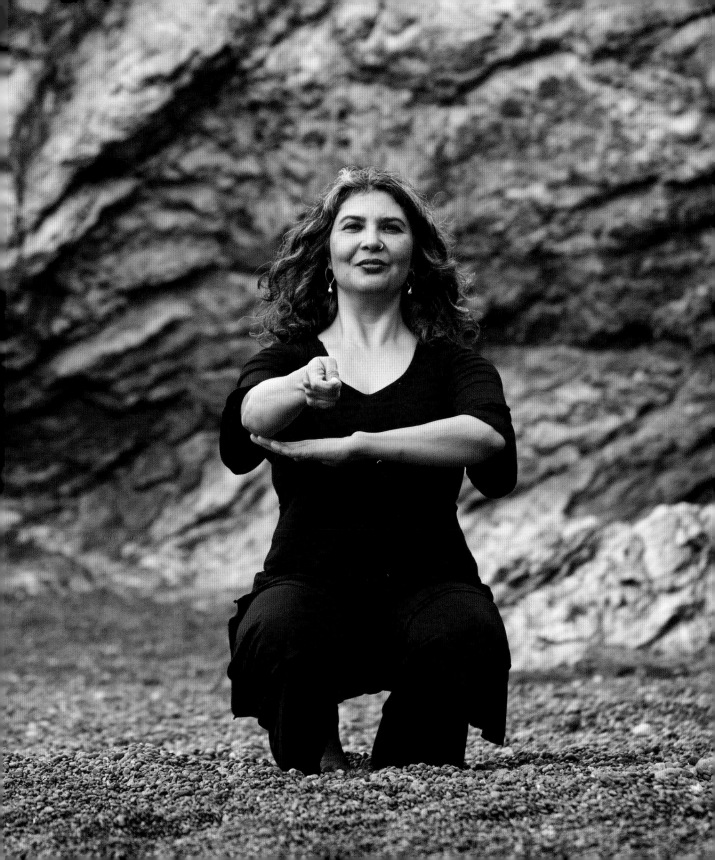

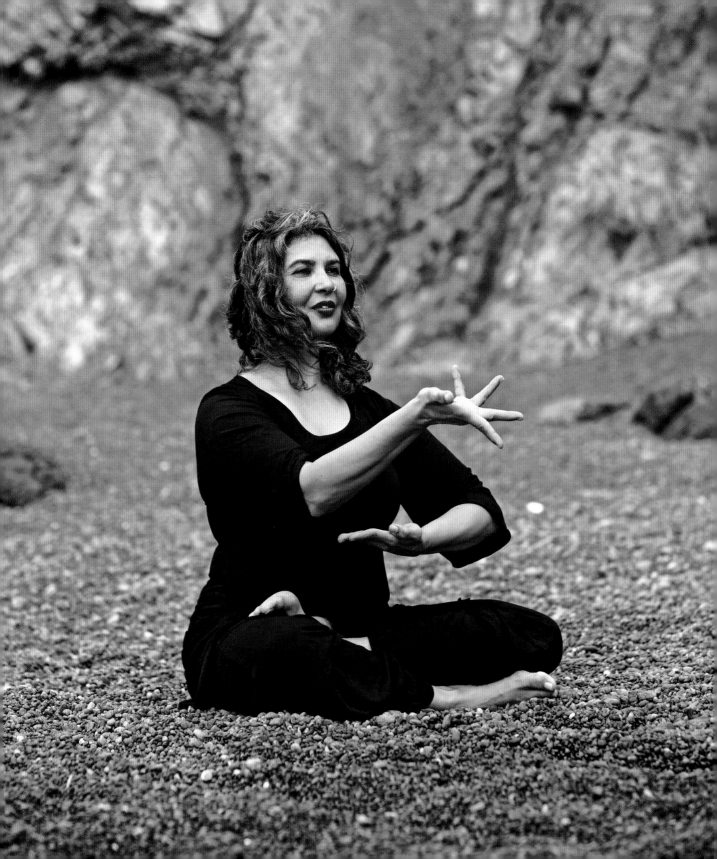

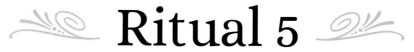

Ritual 5
Akasha, the ether element
Ardha padmanasana with *alapadma mudra*

Mudra

In this pose, *alapadma* represents a lotus flower being offered. Open your fingers like petals in such a way that the fingers are straight, and from the index to the little finger, the fingers separate to create a round shape.

Asana

Sit either on the floor or with your hips elevated on a blanket. Cross the right leg in front of the hips while placing the top of the left foot on the upper right thigh. I suggest you place the right foot under the left knee and switch sides on different days, sometimes having the right foot on top and other times the left.

Ritual

Salutations to the ether element and salutations to she who is the void of space and the voice of the world:

> *"With gratitude in my heart for the blessing of becoming and for the certainty of returning, I take refuge on your ethereal lap, oh Mother, and I ask you to please whisper your messages to me and allow me to foresee what you want me to manifest."*

To the ether element, I offer a flower, or *poola*.

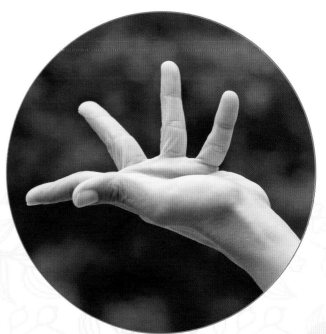

Meditative Yoga

Honoring our inner life

In this section of the practice, we will sit in meditation and contemplation and hold our asana with its corresponding mudra for a longer period of time—a minimum of five to twenty minutes. If you have experience with a personal meditation practice, you can choose to maintain the pose for longer, but if you are new to meditation, increase the time slowly, always choosing to prop your physical body if needed.

The emphasis with this set of ten poses is to deepen our relationship with each one of the mudras that is offered and take inspiration from its unique source—to become one with the symbolism of the mudra. So, although I suggest a different seated pose for each mudra, you could certainly mix-match the seated positions or even sit on a chair.

Dharana means "concentration," and it is the bridge to dhyana, or meditation. It is a yogic technique that will allow you to connect to the depth and mystery of each given symbol. When you concentrate on a seal for a long enough period of time, that seal will reveal its powers to you. Mysteries can be unveiled to us via these sacred emblems and through the awakening of intuition and wisdom. To comprehend the world of symbols as doorways to revelations, we need to be able to perceive beyond our intellectual minds. We must have faith in the methods that have been passed down to us by wise and ancient seers and enter this journey into the unknown with our minds focused and our inner ears and eyes opened wide. The mudras will be the object of our meditation and a key to opening a state of meditation.

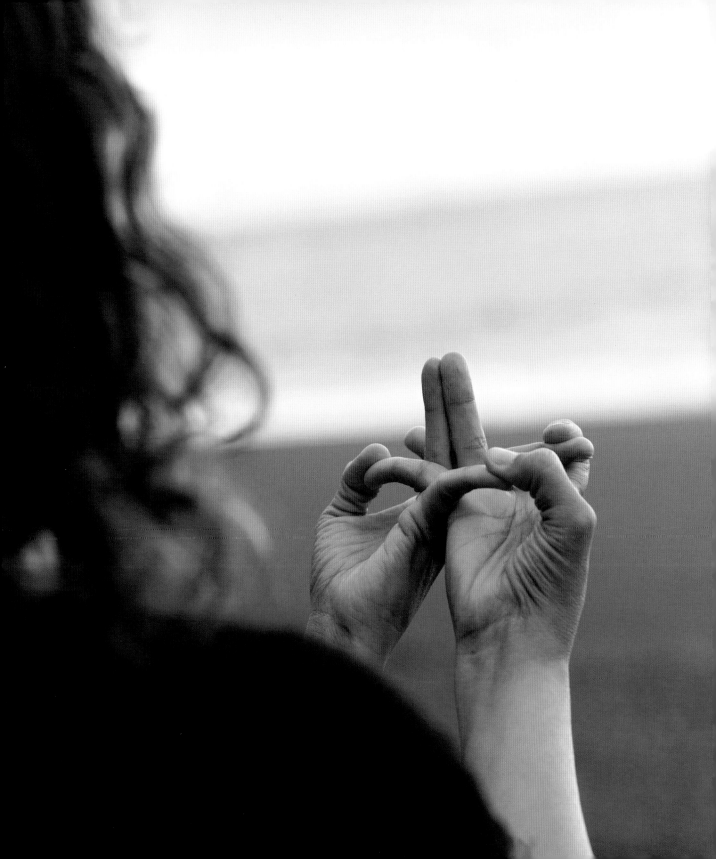

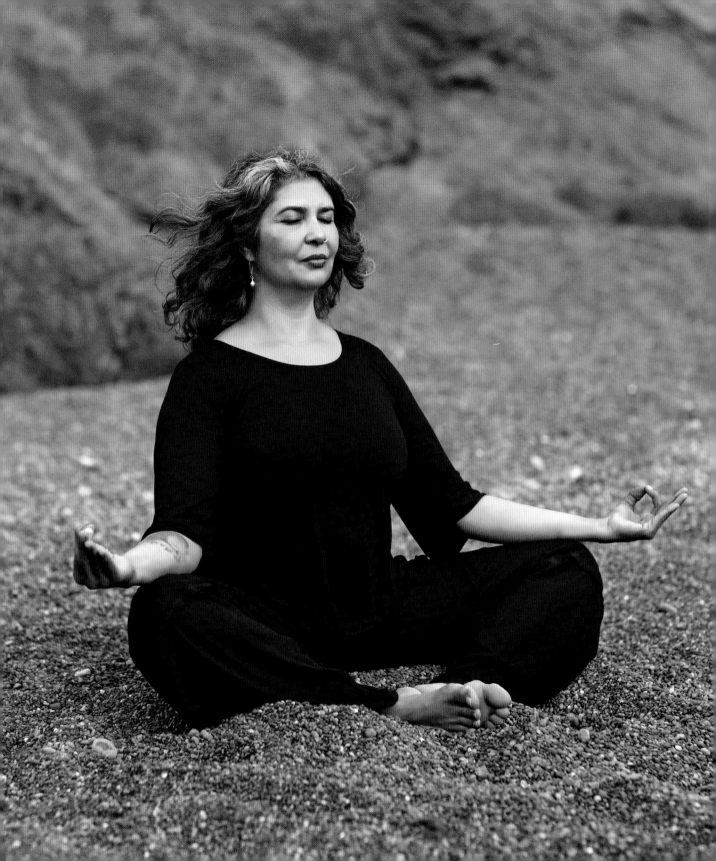

Meditation 1

Bhadrasana, auspicious pose, with *jnana mudra*, wisdom hand gesture

Mudra

Allow your thumb and index finger to touch, and rest your awareness on the energy that is being created within the circle of the two connected fingers. This circle, created with the fingers, can be seen as the ether element yantra: the sacred geometry of the sun and the full moon. The mudra supports us in elevating our minds to reach for our highest potential. This wisdom seal places in our palms the goal of becoming whole and complete.

Asana

Sit comfortably by bringing the soles of your feet together, and move your feet about 10 to 12 inches away from your hips. Press the inner heels and the balls of the big toes together as you find firmness in the legs. Position the shoulders above the sitting bones, and relax the shoulders. Align the back of the head and sacrum. Move the shoulders back while placing your hands or forearms on your knees with the hands in *jnana mudra*. Calling upon the wisdom of your heart to open up to the auspiciousness and benevolence of the sacred beings, begin to focus your attention to the spaciousness of the heart center, and through your hands, visualize that you are attracting the rays of the sun to the center of your chest. Let your breath be free, and focus on the awakening of your inner wisdom and love.

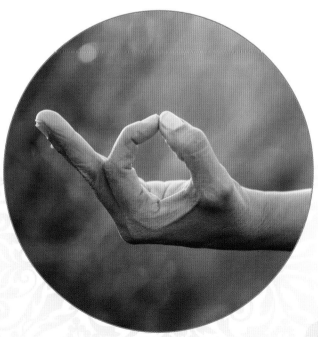

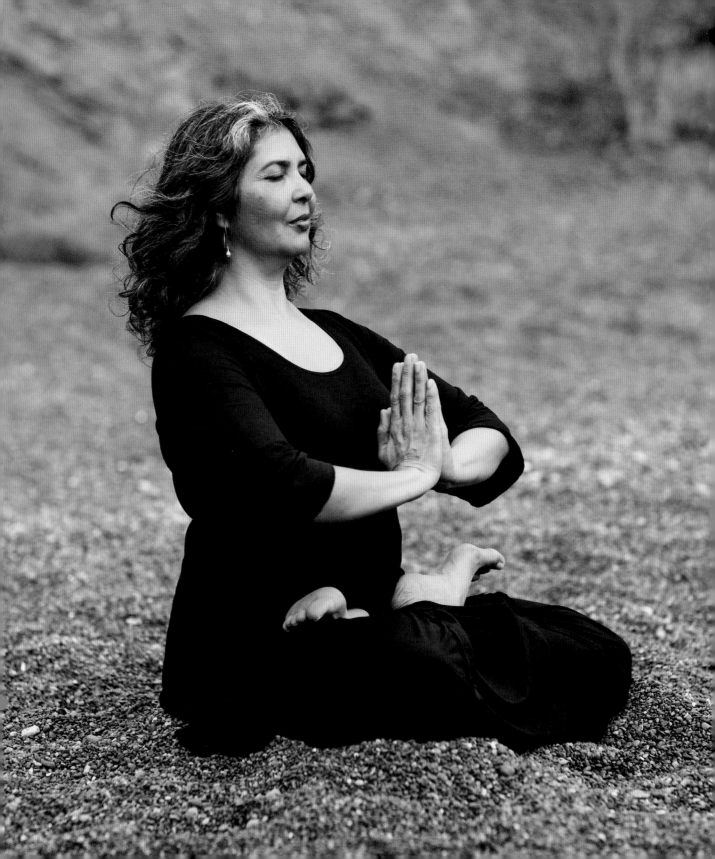

Meditation 2

Padmasana, lotus pose, with *anjali mudra*, prayer hand gesture

Mudra

Anjali mudra is part of so many traditions and awakens the qualities of peace, introspection, respect, and humility within oneself and others. When uniting your palms in front of the heart, you will notice that there are two different ways of making the hand gesture: Hold your fingers pointing up and connecting with your inner guru, God, or both, and the second is to have your fingers pointing forward, dedicating your prayers to the space and the sentient beings around you. These two different ways of forming the prayer hand gesture can be done as a way to respectfully connect with the Divine or with one's immediate surroundings.

Asana

Sit on the floor, and gently bring the outer edge of the right foot to the top of the left thigh. With the left ankle, place the top of the left foot over the right thigh. In *padmasana*, the soles of the feet are turned toward the sky. This pose can be substituted with *sukhasana*, a simple and easy cross-legged position. With the hands in prayer, you are inviting any opposing tendencies of the heart and all that appears to be separated to come together to support your spirit to soar in prayer and in dedication.

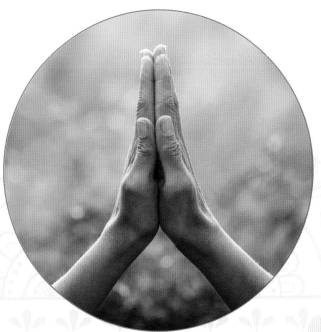

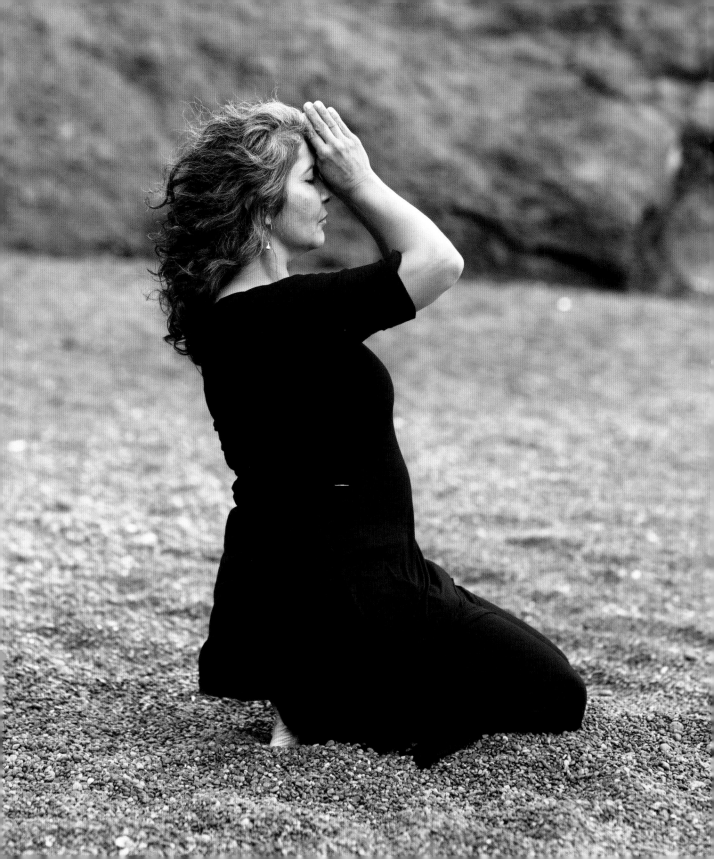

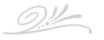

Meditation 3

Prajapasana, praying pose, with *kapota mudra*

Mudra

We can begin this hand gesture with our hands in prayer. Then, by keeping the tip of the fingers and the palms of the hands together, separate the space between your hands creating a cave within your palms. As you create a diamond-like shape with your hands and place your hands on your forehead, you can open you inner vision to all the possibilities that could be made available to you. You can lower your hands in *kapota* to your heart center and ask for divine light to open your heart and purify your actions. *Kapota* in the *Abhinayadarpanam* text is translated as a salutation, and it is considered a way to respectfully address another being.

Asana

Prajapa means "to pray." Kneeling with your toes tucked under, sit on your heels. Align the sitting bones with the heels and sit upright. Place your hands in *kapota mudra*, and position them before the third eye, in between your eyebrows. Concentrate on the *ajna* chakra, the center of intuition and wisdom within the body, and visualize the mudra shining a special clearing light over your mind. Pray for purity of thought and clarity of mind. If you wish, in addition to asana and mudra, you can add the vocalization of the bija mantra, *om*, and resound it a few times. The *om* sound stimulates the *ajna* chakra.

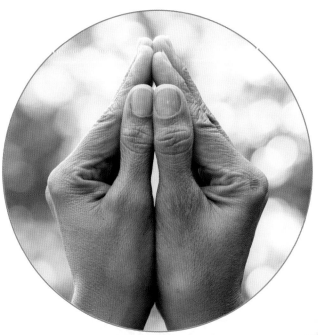

Meditation 4

Siddhasana, the realized one pose, with *Bhairava mudra*

Mudra

Place the back of the right hand on top of the left hand. The fingers should remain together but relaxed. Notice that the thumbs are touching the base of the index fingers. With everyone, the right side of the body represents the masculine, the solar side. In this meditative mudra, we have the male energy of Lord Shiva as the lead with his counterpart Shakti placed below.

Shiva in his fearful aspect of Bhairava empowers us to be fearless, and he and only he has the power to annihilate evil, deeply rooted impressions upon our psyche. He is our protector. While meditating on this mudra, you can whisper the mantra, "*om namah Shivaya*," meaning, "I surrender myself to Shiva."

Asana

In this simplified version of *siddhasana*, place your left heel in front of the pubic bone and cross your right leg in front of your body while placing the outer edge of the right foot in the fold between your left calf and left thigh. Sit upright and stay balanced. With the hands in *Bhairava mudra*, evoke the power of Shiva in his fierce manifestation. Sit still and focus on your hands. Visualize an amber light shinning in your hands like a sacred fire. Begin to offer your thoughts, memories, and emotions into Shiva's sacrificial fire of transformation and purification.

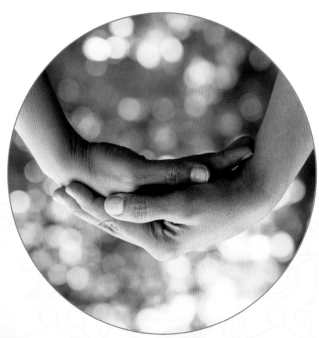

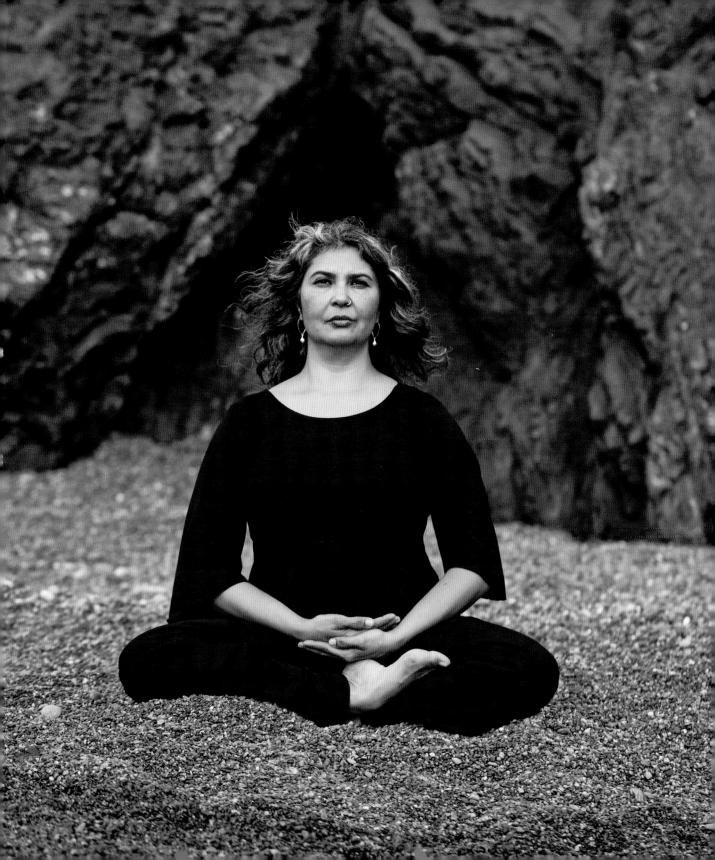

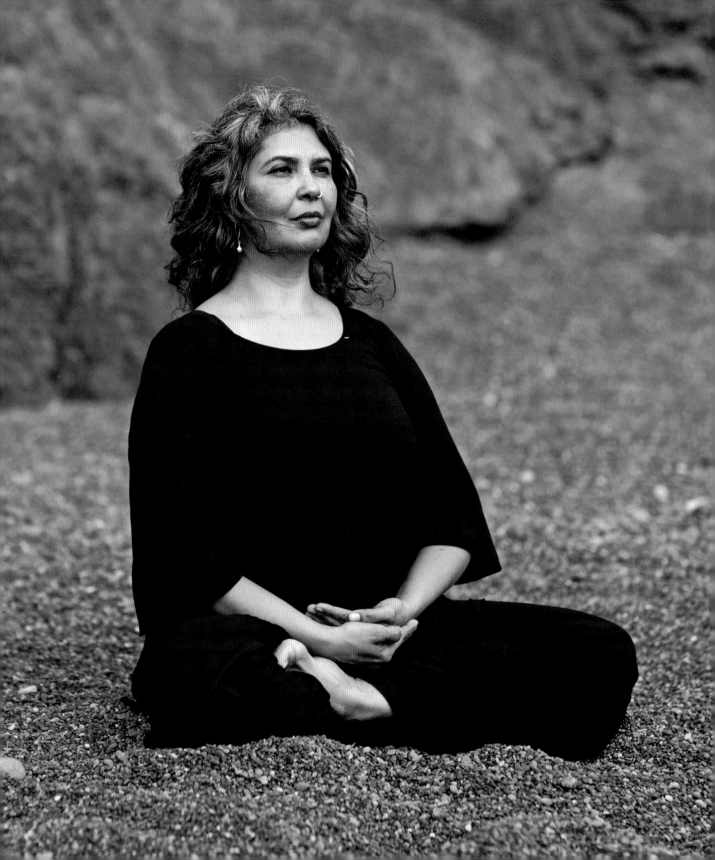

Meditation 5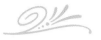

Siddha yoni asana, the powerful source pose,
with *Bhairavi mudra*

Mudra

Place the back of the left hand on top of the right palm. The thumbs will be touching the base of the index fingers, and your hands will become a bowl-like recipient. The left side of the body represents the feminine, the lunar side, and in this meditative mudra we are appreciative of having the female energy of Shakti guiding and controlling our inner winds and *pranic* force. Shakti is life force, activation, and protection.

While contemplating this mudra, reflect on the presence of her sustaining force within you, and if you wish, vocalize her syllable mantra, "*Hreem.*"

Asana

Seated on the floor, place your right heel in front of the pubic bone, cross your left leg in front of your body, and place the outer edge of the left foot in the fold between your right calf and thigh. As you do this, find equilibrium and ground yourself through the hips.

Place your hands in *Bhairavi mudra* and evoke the power of Shakti in one of her most intense and benevolent forms. Bhairavi is considered to be one of the ten Mahavidyas, or aspects of wisdom, that brings forth insight and spiritual knowledge in the form of revelation. While sitting still and focusing on your hands, visualize a red upside-down triangle balancing in the center of your palms. This triangle encapsulates the power of the feminine. With concentration, direct your mind's heart unto this symbol, and pray to receive her empowerment.

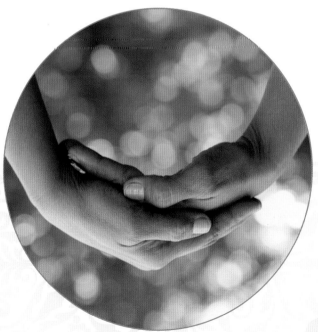

Meditation 6

Vajrasana, thunderbolt pose, with hridaya mudra

Mudra

Hridaya mudra means "heart gesture." Open your palms and fingers. Begin by bringing the tips of the index fingers to the bases of the thumbs, creating a spiral-like shape with your index fingers. Then, connect the middle and ring fingers to the thumb, stretching the little finger away from the other fingers. Meditating on this hand gesture, open your heart and enter into the inner sanctum of your soul.

Asana

While kneeling, come to sit on your heels with the tops of your feet touching the ground. If you need, place a blanket under your feet or your hips. Sit upright and move your chest up, further out than your head.

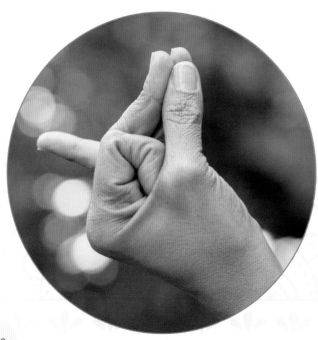

Bring your hands into the heart seal, either by lifting your hands to chest height or by resting the backs of your hands on your lap. This mudra invites you to be present in the spaciousness of your heart center.

With clear intention to awaken the qualities of the heart, concentrate your mind on the inevitable winds of change, on the natural cycles of expansion and contraction, and on the spiritual force that resides within us all. This concentration might awaken sensations, feelings, and memories, and you can use this opportunity to openly receive and willingly offer each one of them. Clearing the mirror of the heart requires effort and surrender like any other spiritual practice.

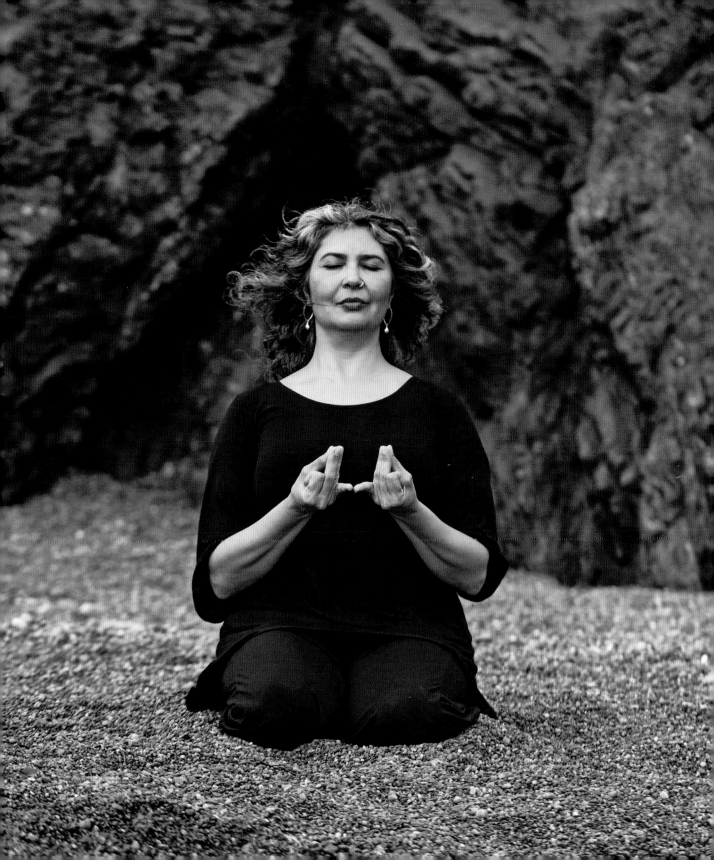

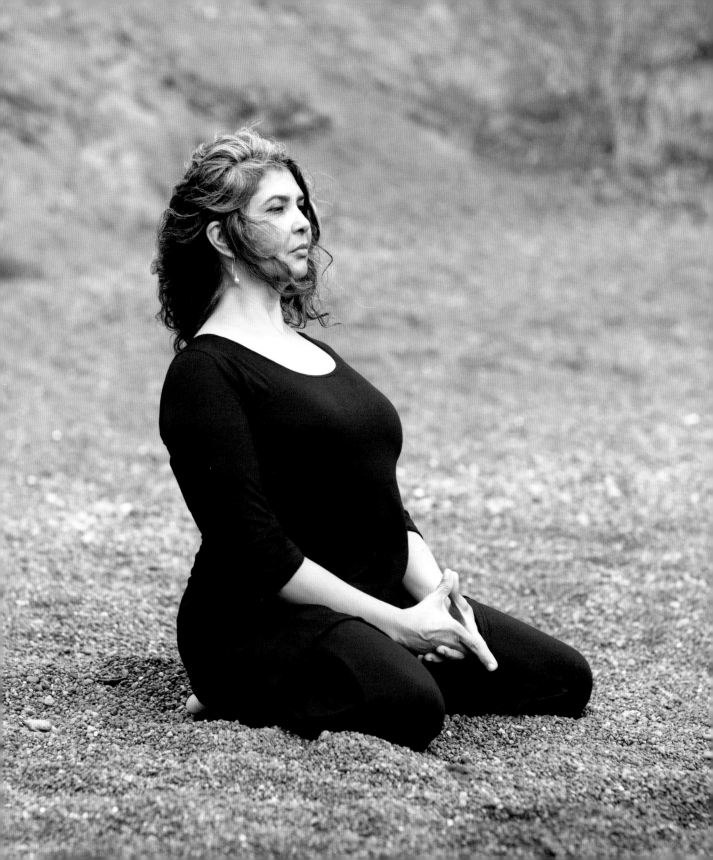

Meditation 7

Ghantasana, bell pose, with *yoni mudra*

Mudra

Turn your palms up and move your fingers forward, interlocking them. Stretch the index fingers forward, and bring them to touch. Stretch the thumbs toward your heart, and bring them to touch, creating the shape of a water drop in your hands.

Yoni is usually descriptive of the female organ of generation and symbolizes the energy of creation. Still, the word can also mean "descent," "source," "womb," or "water."

Point your index fingers down and your thumbs up, and begin to breath. As you inhale, bring the power of the earth to your heart through your mudra. As you exhale, imagine a stream of cleansing water-like light flowing downstream from your heart toward your hands and into the womb of the earth. Invite the stability of the earth while breathing in, and wash away impurities while breathing out.

Asana

Start on hands and knees and unite your big toes as you separate your knees wider than the hips. Sit back on your heels, keeping the knees open like the opening of a bell. This pose allows for a feeling of release toward the earth. Gently lift your heart and relax your shoulders. Bring your hands to *yoni mudra*, or the feminine source mudra, and rest your arms as you place your hands between your thighs. Concentrate on your hands and on the power of creation of this symbol while calling upon the attributes of the feminine that you would like to attain.

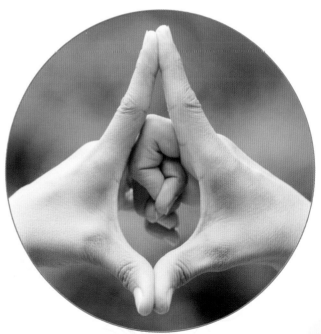

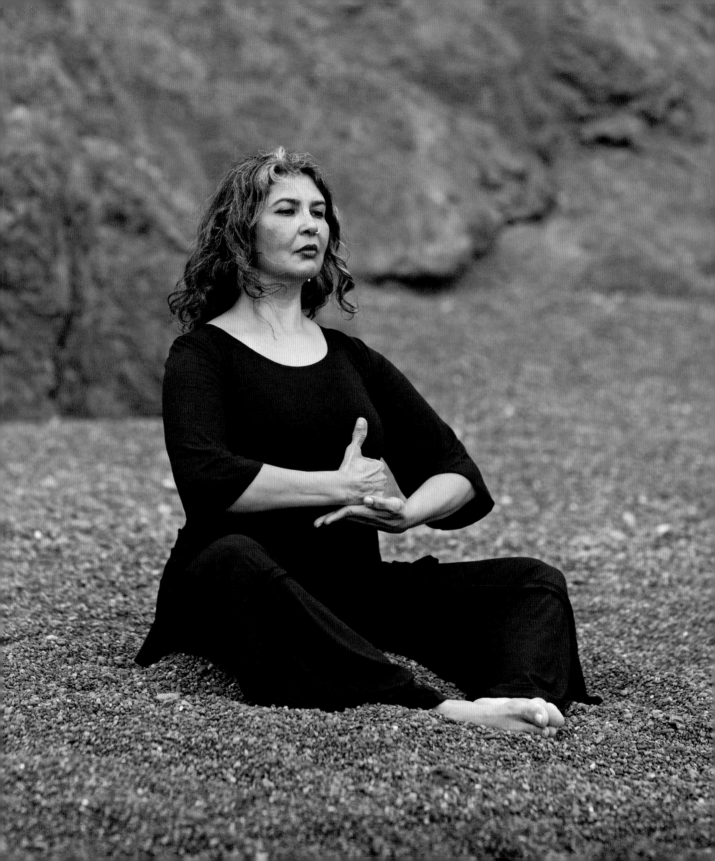

Meditation 8

Baddha konasana with *yoni-lingam mudra*

Mudra

Place your right hand in *sikhara*, right thumb up and the other fingers make a fist-like base for the thumb. Position on top of the left hand in *pataka mudra*, flat palm with fingers together, forming *yoni-lingam mudra*.

Stay relaxed and in deep concentration while sitting upright. Keep a soft gaze, and begin to notice your spontaneous exhalation. With each exhalation, you can choose to say the mantra: "*swaha,*" or "I surrender." Clearing old impressions and opening up to create something new within your psyche, shift your inner gaze to the mudra, and begin to inquire about the potential of creation within you. Be attentive to unveiling what might be covering your ability to see what you need to see, do what you need to do, and bring what you need to bring into existence. Focus on your goal, and ask for guidance with the actions you need to take to manifest change.

Asana

In this variation of *baddha konasana*, sit on the ground, bring the soles of your feet together, and move your feet away from your hips about 18 inches or so, giving yourself a bigger foundation.

The *yoni-lingam mudra* symbolizes the sacred union between Shiva and Shakti, and it guides us into uniting the opposites within ourselves. Meditate on the power of creation that happens through the union of the individual soul with the universal soul. You may want to whisper the mantra *"om Shiva, om Shakti, namah Shiva, namah Shakti."*

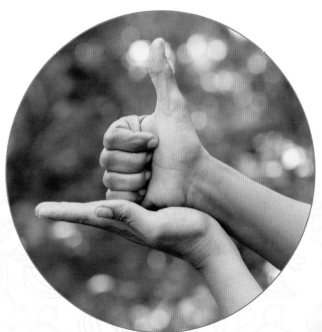

Meditation 9

Sukhasana, easy cross-legged position,
with *mandala mudra*, offering hand gesture

Mudra

Open your hands with palms facing up, and interlock the four fingers from little to index. Bring your thumbs to touch the pads of the little fingers, and bring your index fingers to the pads of your middle fingers. Lastly, stretch the ring fingers out while uniting them and moving the tips of your ring fingers upward.

The *mandala* hand gesture is a microcosmic representation of the macrocosmic universe. The upward ring fingers depict Mount Meru, and the other four points depict the four main directions and the sun and the moon. Symbolically, Mount Meru relates to the spine in our bodies, the four regions are our four limbs, and the sun and the moon are our eyes. This mudra originates from the Tibetan Buddhist tradition, so offer your prayers to all the Buddhas so that they may purify the world.

Asana

Begin by sitting with your hips elevated by a blanket, and cross your left leg in front of the right leg. Rest your heels under the opposite shin bones, supporting the knees by allowing them to be higher than the ground level. The name of this pose suggests the mood that we are intending to achieve internally, namely, a state of ease.

While holding the *mandala mudra*, we are going to vocalize a mantra for universal peace, singing it over the mudra as a blessing to all sentient beings: *"Om bishwa shanti ananda."* It means, "May there be universal peace and bliss forever." This prayer is from T.Y.S. Lama Gangchen.

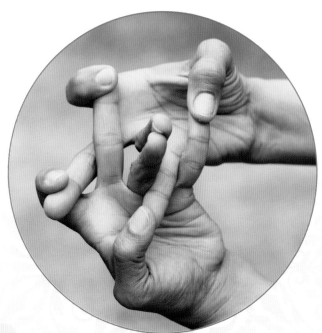

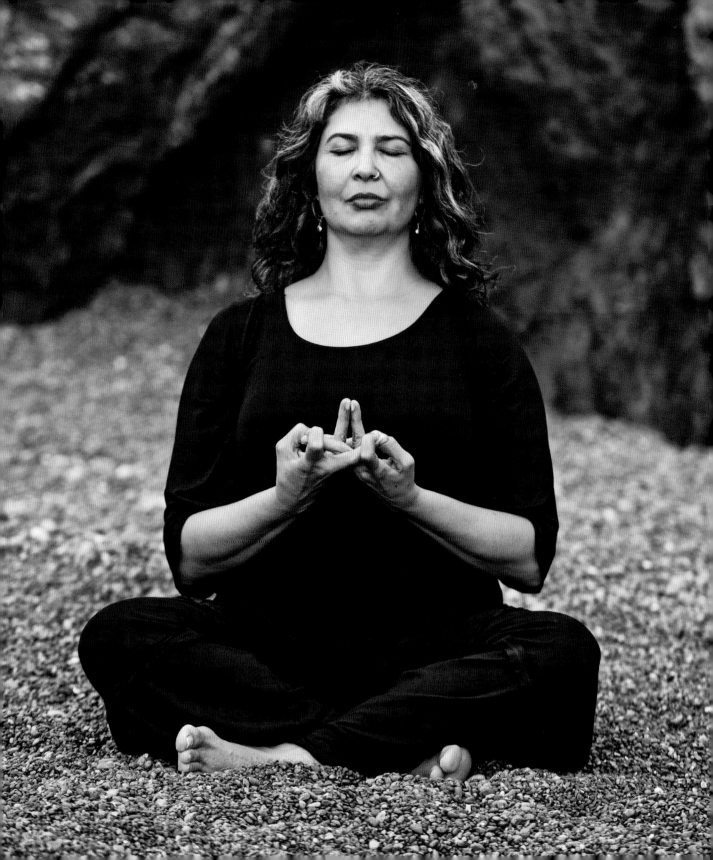

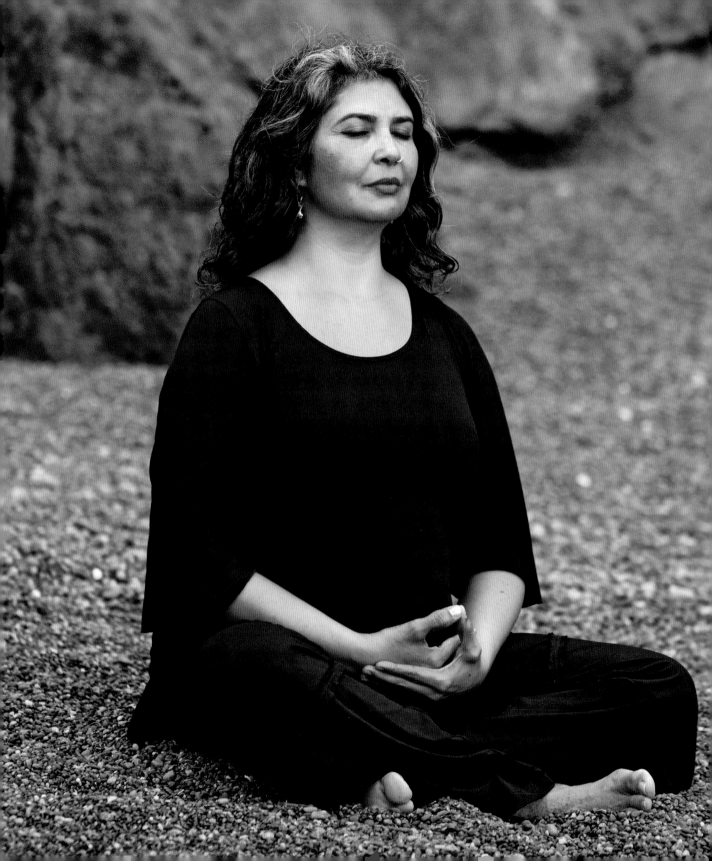

Meditation 10

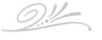

Sukhasana, easy cross-legged position, with dhyana mudra, meditation hand gesture

Mudra

Place the back of the right hand on top of the left palm, and create the shape of a bowl with your hands. Now, bring the thumbs to touch, creating a circle between your thumbs and index fingers. I would like for us to focus on *dhyana mudra* as has been shown as the *Buddha Shakyamuni mudra*. While the hand gesture is the same, in our mind's heart, we are calling and connecting to the presence of Buddha and focusing on our potential to reach enlightenment in this life. The circle you form with your thumbs represents the wheel of dharma and samsara. To be able to cross this ocean of material suffering, we ask for the guidance of Guru Buddha Shakyamuni while chanting, *"Om muni muni maha muni Shakyamuni soha,"* which means, "Oh wise, great wise Shakyamuni, I offer myself onto you."

Asana

Begin by sitting with your hips elevated, and cross your right leg in front of the left leg, resting your heels under the opposite chin bones, establishing firmness and ease.

Bring your hands to the meditation hand gesture, and as you unite the right and left thumbs, activate the central line of energy or *sushumna nadi* in your awareness, and in silence make a vow to realign with your soul's purpose in this life.

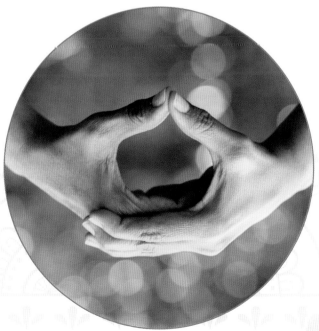

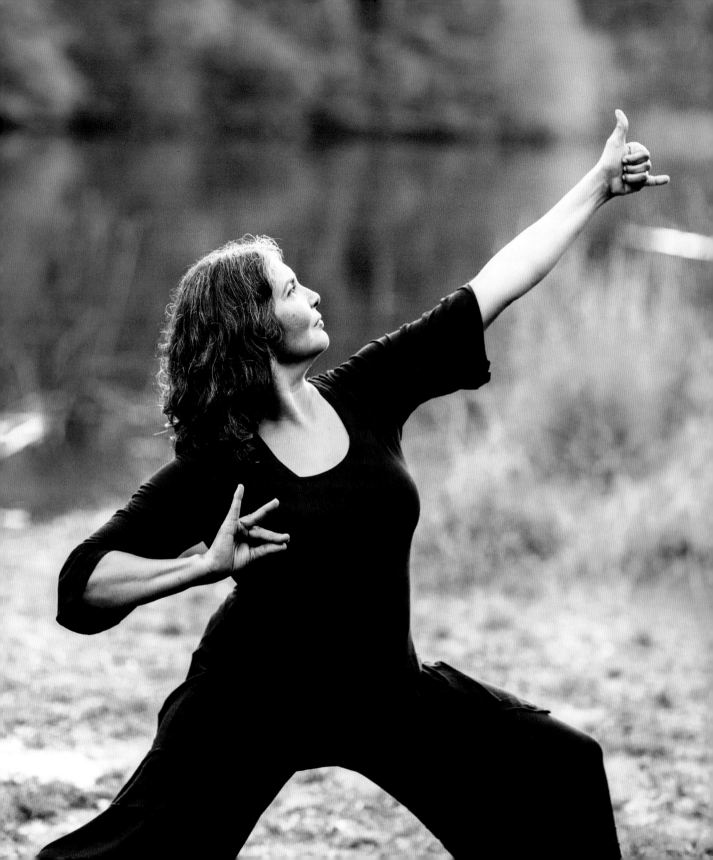

Yoga Bijasanas and Mudrasanas

Honoring the self, the creation, and the deities

In this larger part of the book, we will experiment with poses and hand gestures that give shape to our devotional practice or that support our effort to embody our Bhakti. This sadhana will work on increasing resilience and balance, while evoking through yoga the power and the grace of nature and the Divine. Notice that most of the poses need balance, so practice these combinations on both sides.

While holding the poses offered in this part of the book, be attentive to your breathing. You can either simply observe the natural flow of the breath, or engage with the fullness of the in breath and the completeness of the out breath. The body is being moved by prana, and this vital life force is coming from the spirit's world, which we want to stay tuned to during this practice.

We will hold the poses in this section for five to ten cycles of breath, or two to three minutes. The focus on our breath awakens our gratitude for being alive and supports our prayers and our intention as we hold these combinations of asana and mudra.

Remember, the bijasanas contain the seed power of the deities, and the mudrasanas contain the keys to the elements that you are evoking.

Pose 1

Kalpavrikshasana, wish-fulfilling tree pose,
with *sarva mangala mudra*

Mudra

This mudra, like *varada mudra*, is a hand gesture of granting blessings. *Sarva* means "universe" and *mangala* means "prosperity"; *sarva mangala* means to wish auspiciousness for all. Bring your hands above your head, and with your fingers placed together, make a shallow bowl-like shape with your hands. Bring them close to each other with your palms facing forward.

Asana

Start by pressing your feet firmly on the ground, rooting through the four corners of your feet, the inner and outer heels, the mounds of your big and little toes. Spread the roots of the left foot wider, and lift your right foot to place the sole of your right foot on either your left inner shin or left inner thigh. Balance on your left foot while keeping the back of the body in alignment. Open your arms to the sides, inhaling all the blessings and gifts you have in your hands, and place your hands in the *sarva mangala mudra*. Voice a prayer blessing for auspiciousness for others. Feel in your heart that your prayer is meaningful and that it makes a difference in bringing your light to the world.

Kalpavriksha is a wish-fulfilling tree and a bountiful gift giver. Special types of trees in India have received this name because of the precious gifts that they have shared, the shelter they give, and the unique spiritual nourishment they offer. Take a stand and be generous.

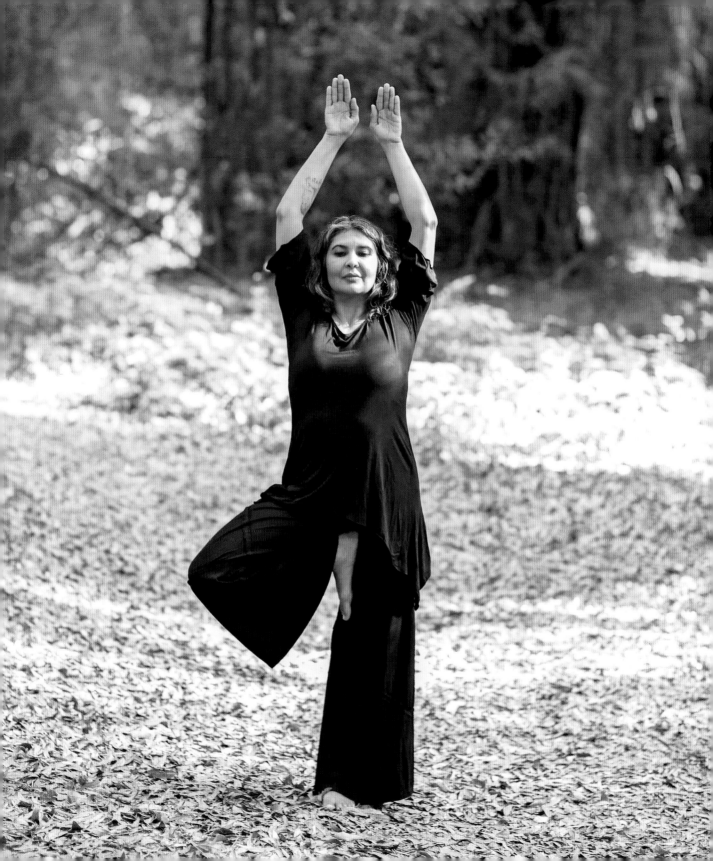

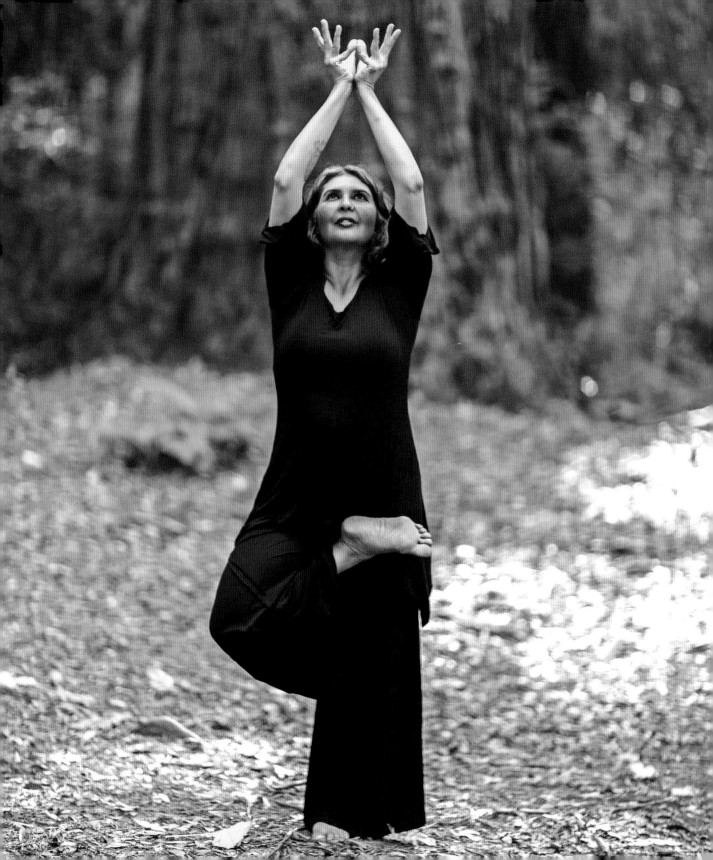

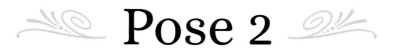

Pose 2

Ardha padma vrikshasana with *padma mudra*

Mudra

Bring your hands together in prayer by adopting the *anjali mudra* in front of the heart, and look to the hands. Keep the wrists, thumbs, and little fingers together while separating the index, middle, and ring fingers, moving them away from the palm and opening them like a flower. As you inhale, begin to move your prayer up, and slowly open it into a lotus hand gesture, *padma mudra*, above your head. You can look straight ahead or shift the gaze up if you can remain balanced and connected to the earth through your feet. Reflect on the purity of your heart, and make a wish that your prayers may come into full bloom.

As you stay with one foot on the ground and the other pointing skyward, remember both of your missions—the spiritual and the human—while keeping your attention and gaze on your prayer. May your dreams come true.

Asana

Stand balanced on both feet in *samasthiti*, or equal standing. Balance on your left foot, and bring the top of the right foot toward the left hip. Pushing the left knee down and pressing the top of the right foot against the left thigh, define your balance by focusing on the central line of your body, along your spine.

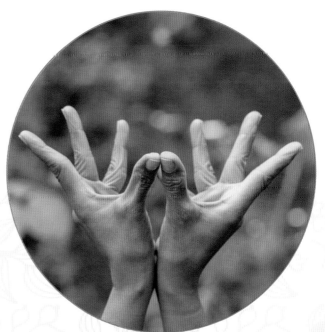

Pose 3

Ganesha bijasana, mandala pada asana
with two hands in *kapittha mudra*

Mudra

Put your thumbs up, and bring the tops of your index fingers to rest on the tops of the thumbs. Keep the hands active but soft. *Kapittha* is used for many different poses, has many meanings, and can be used in multiple ways.

In *hastabhinaya, kapittha mudra* it is not specifically the *Ganesha mudra*, though it is used to show one of Ganesha's attributes: his lasso of mercy.

Asana

Stand tall and separate your feet at least 20 inches apart. Turn your toes and knees out while bending the knees. Ground yourself through the center of the heels, point your knees to your toes, and align the back of your head with the sacrum, so the back of the body is leaning against an imaginary wall. Keep your shoulders relaxed while bending the elbows to bring your hands in *kapittha* near your hips, with your thumbs pointing down.

The big stances in *mandala pada* represent Ganesha's big body or *maha kaya*. The *kapittha* hands show us the lasso-like rope, or *pasha*, that Ganesha uses as an instrument to pull the devotees back onto the path of grace and dharma. Hold this pose for a long period of time, feeling the blessing and presence of Lord Ganesha.

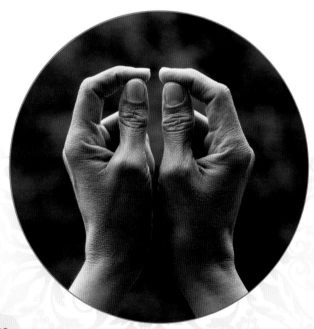

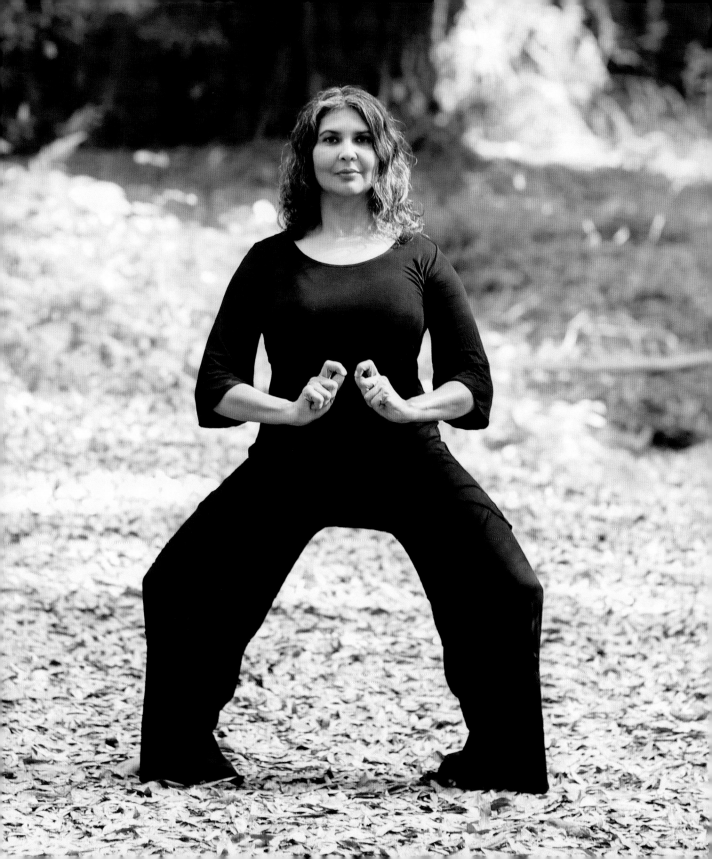

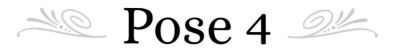

Pose 4

Nritya Ganesha or dancing Ganesha, *nupura pada asana* with two hands in *pataka mudra*

Mudra

Pataka hasta, or flat palms, is used to show the playing of the drum. Flatten your palms and bend your wrists so that the wrists are moving in while the fingertips are moving out, creating a sharp angle on the wrists. Relax your shoulders and open your elbows sideways to bring the beauty of Odissi to this pose.

Asana

This is a storytelling asana. Like his father, Shiva, Ganesha is also depicted as a dancer and a musician. While dancing, Ganesha plays his drum, the *dolak*, and in ecstasy he celebrates life with his devotees. Because Ganesha has traveled into the realm of death, after his father Shiva initiated him in the mysteries of dying, Ganesha knows how life is precious and takes any opportunity he has to celebrate life.

Stand tall with your feet together, like in the mountain pose. Open your feet out as you begin to bend your knees. Now, transfer the weight of your body to your left foot while moving your right foot forward, opening your right knee out and pointing your right foot to the earth. If you were looking at this shape sideways, you would see that the right leg is on a three-dimensional plane. This is to accommodate the drum on your lap. Stay still and stand joyfully in this asana.

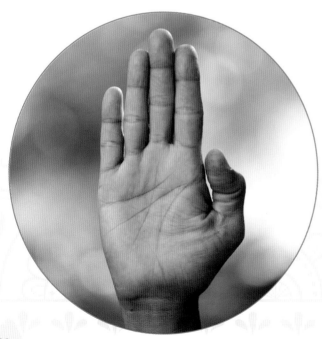

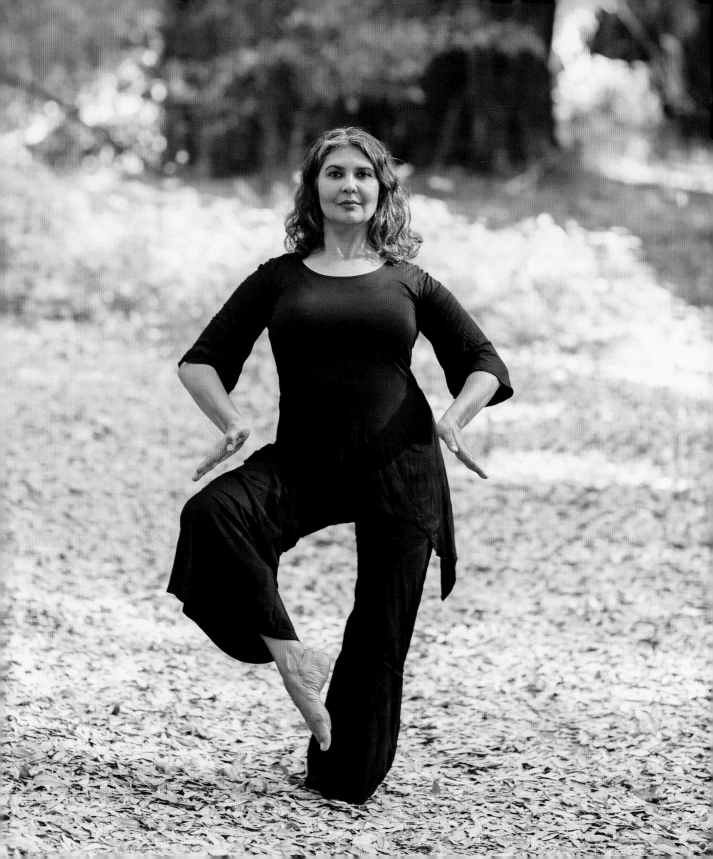

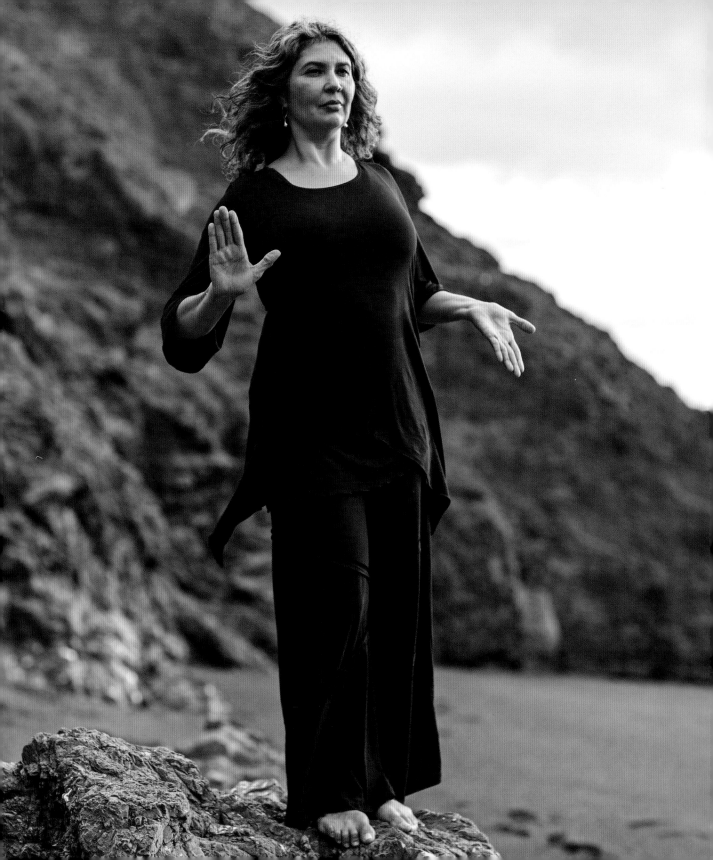

Pose 5

Parvati bijasana, abhanga asana with right hand in *abhaya mudra* and left hand in *varada mudra*

Mudras

Abhaya, or "without fear," is a mudra that provides protection and guardianship. Simply hold the right hand in front of your body with palm facing forward and fingers pointing up to the sky. The heel of your right hand will move forward to be aligned with the fingers pointing up. Hold your ground and your boundaries.

Varada, or "blessing," is a mudra that shows generosity and abundance. Open your left palm and have it facing forward with your fingers pointing down. Move the heel of your left hand forward to align with the tips of the fingers, and allow your heart's treasures to flow downstream to your palms.

These two hand gestures can be used separately or in combination, and they are shared among many deities.

In the tradition of Odissi, both *abhaya* and *varada* are shown with the thumbs open in *ardhachandra*, the half-moon hand gesture.

Asana

Stand tall with feet parallel and close together. Bend your right knee without lifting your right heel, and let the hips naturally shift to the left. Bring your hands to *abhaya* on the right and *varada* on the left, and open yourself to feel Parvati Devi's presence.

Parvati is the daughter of the mountain, and she has the fragrance of the earth. Beloved of Shiva, mother of Ganesha and Skanda, and a perfected yogini, she bestows her blessings of firmness and realization onto her children and devotees.

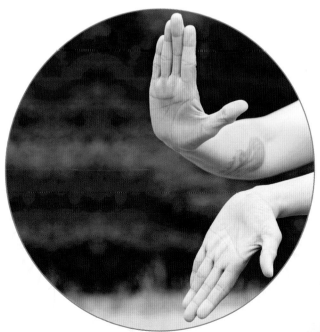

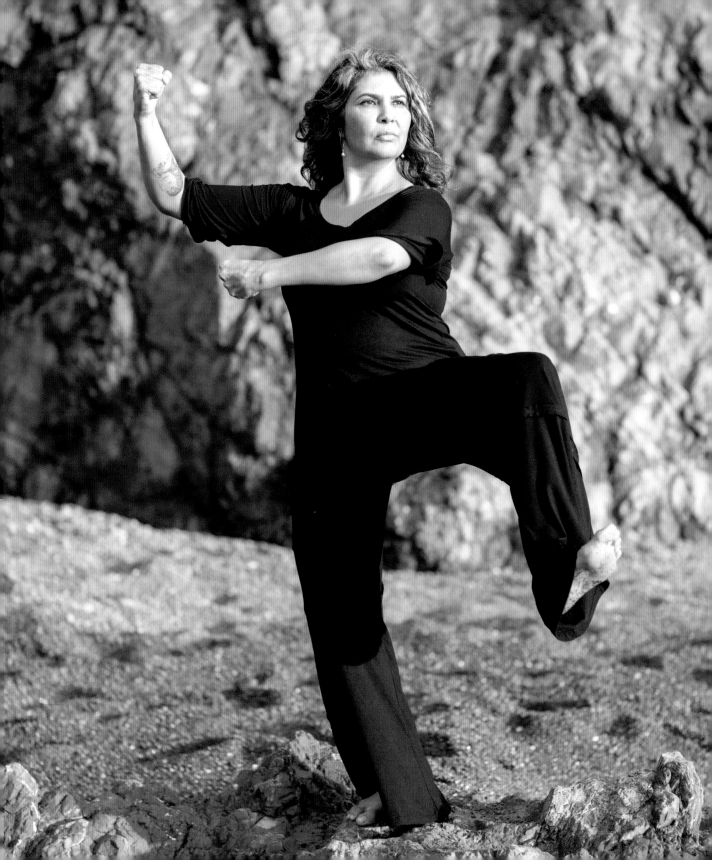

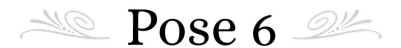

Pose 6

Shakti bijasana, uttolita pada asana with *musti mudra*

Mudra

Musti literally means "fist." Simply close your fingers, and make a fist with your hands—it symbolizes strength and power.

Asana

Shakti is the feminine power principle. In her glory and grace, she shows us our latent potential as she herself resides within our bodies as a powerful force called Kundalini Shakti.

In this abhinaya, Devi is aroused and ready to fight in order to protect her children. She is holding the trisula, or trident, and she is ready to pierce and destroy evil in the form of ignorance. Her power and protection is a model for us, orienting us on the important mission of taking care of each other and increasing morality and goodness. Jai Ma!

Begin by standing tall with feet one hip apart.

Turn your toes and knees out, and begin to bend your knees to a comfortable and firm level. Bring your hands to *musti mudra*, and hold the hands in front of the heart to start.

Shift the weight to your right foot, and begin to balance on that side while lifting your left foot to knee height. Move your hands to the right so the right elbow is aligned with the right shoulder and the right hand is higher than the elbow. Move your left hand and arm to the right to be slightly below the heart. Shift your gaze over to the left, and be ready. Just in case it is needed.

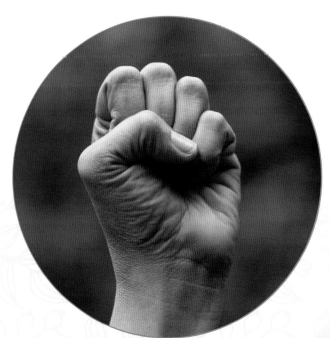

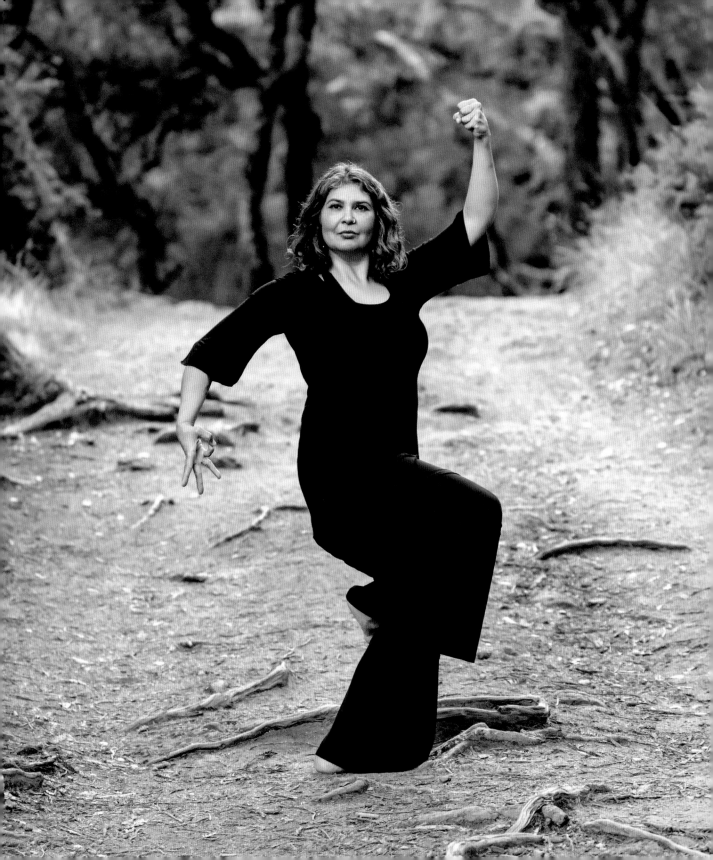

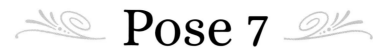

Pose 7

Durga bijasana, bandhani pada asana with *musti* and *trisula mudras*

Mudras

For the trident hand gesture, simply connect the thumb to the little finger, and open the three central fingers of your hand away from each other. The trident is a powerful weapon, a gift from Siva himself to Parvati. Bringing into balance the qualities of nature—perfection (sattva guna) in the middle, inertia (tamas guna) on the right, and movement (rajas guna) on the left—the trident represents equilibrium that leads to perfection.

For the *musti* hand gesture, as you make a fist, gather your inner strength in your hands and hold on to it tightly.

Asana

In this position, we are telling a specific story of Durga Devi victoriously conquering the demon Mahiṣāsura during the second battle of the Devi Mahatmyam by Sage Markandeya. In this pose, we have the devi stepping over the shoulder of this bull-like demon and piercing him with her trident.

Stand with your feet parallel, and by bending the knees, place the back of your right foot behind the back of the left knee. Sit deeper while pointing both knees forward. Keep your hips square as you add a gentle twist to the right with the upper body. Now add the mudras, with your right hand becoming the trident and your left holding the rod of the trident. Pierce all pride, egocentrism, and greed (within and without).

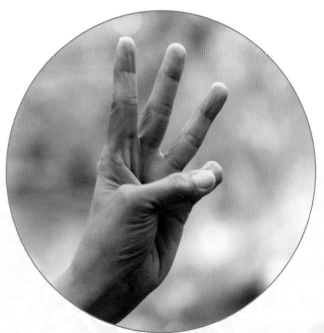

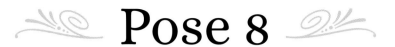

Pose 8

Svastikasana with *svastika mudra*

Mudra

The svastika symbol represents auspiciousness and brings the power of balance. To perform this mudra, you can bring your hands in *pataka*, flat palms, in front of your chest. Make the shape of a cross with your forearms. Press the heels of the hands out, and move the hands away from the chest, creating a vortex of energy in front of the heart.

In this position, the svastika represents stability and prosperity in the heart.

Asana

Sit on the floor and cross your legs such that the feet are flexed and positioned underneath your knees, while forming the shape of the svastika on the lower body. The svastika symbol is associated with the first chakra, with the feminine, and with Ganesha, the remover of obstacles. As you sit firmly in this position, meditate upon blessings of protection and the removal of spiritual blockages.

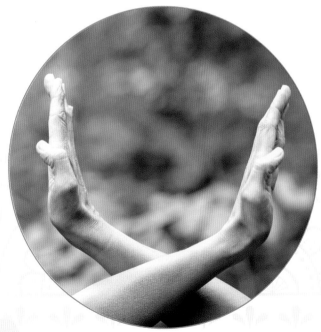

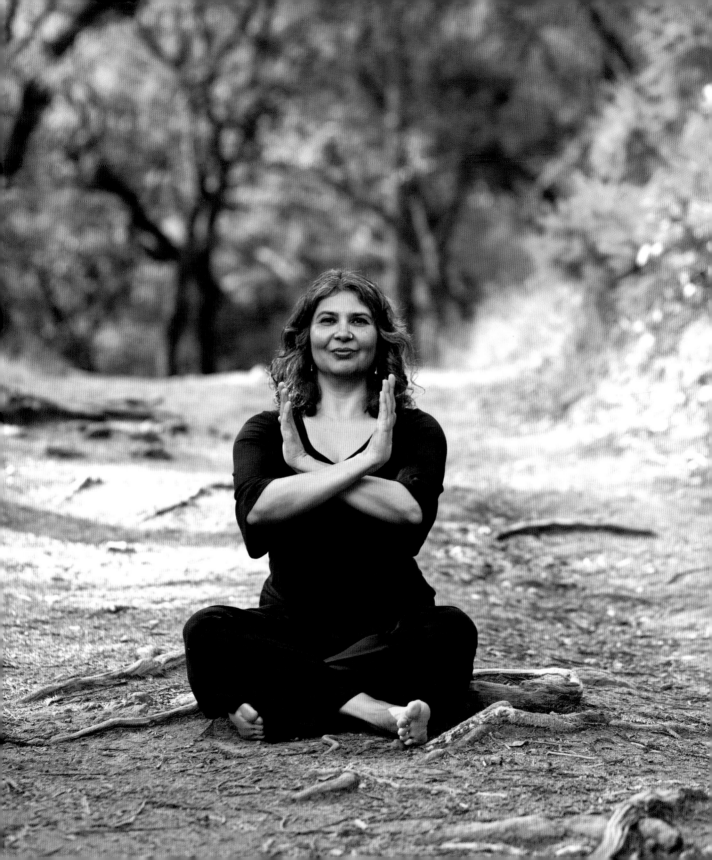

Pose 9

Dola hasta mudra and the Devi text

With the *dola hasta mudra* comes awareness of the feminine. When you see this mudra, you will identify with either a *devi* (a goddess) or a *nata* (a dancer). Bring your awareness to your hands, and by keeping the back of your hands up, bend the wrists while draping the fingers down. The fingers should be together and yet the hands should be relaxed and firm.

Devi, or the Mother Goddess

> *"ya devi sarva bhuteshu matru rupena sansthita namatasyai namastasyai namastasyai namo namaha"*

> *"I bow again and again in reverence to the goddess who is present in every being as Mother."*

The great goddess is known by many names, and as she gives birth to all manifested creation, she becomes the mother of all and she resides within all. We all have within ourselves her strength, her wisdom, and her love. We all have within ourselves her power to transform, create, and sustain. Pervading everything, she keeps the rhythm of the universe in sync with the rhythm of her benevolent heart, propelling us to uncover love for all things and all beings. Connecting with this feminine force, or Shakti, she reveals that maya is a way to tap into her realm and discover hidden abilities that can be used for healing and awakening.

Thinking of the mother as being of three different qualities, we come to the concept of Trimurti, or "the trilogy":

- Sarasvati Devi: the energy of creation,
- Lakshmi Devi: the energy of sustenance, and
- Shakti Devi: the energy of transformation.

These three main aspects of the Devi are the starting point to understanding her thousandfold forms and her unimaginable benevolence.

Sarasvati's masculine counterpart is Lord Brahma, Lakshmi's is Lord Vishnu, and Shakti's is Lord Shiva. Keeping the families together when worshipping them is very important.

Sarasvati and Brahma are associated together but worshipped separately. Other names for Sarasvati are Savitri, meaning "rays of light," Vag Devi, or the goddess of speech, Swaratmika, or the goddess that exists as sound, Sarada, or the goddess of autumn, and Brahmi, meaning "the power of Brahma."

> *"May Sarasvati Devi remain on a lotus at the bottom of my heart and inspire me with her pure springlike waters. May she sit in a lotus at the crown of my head and clear my mind with her waterfall-like blessings. May she sit in her lotus at the tip of my tongue and clear my speech with her wise riverine waters."*

Lakshmi and Vishnu are mainly worshipped as Sri Sri Radha and Krishna, who appeared in this world to reveal the ecstatic love and devotion that they have for each other. Sita and Rama, in turn, appeared in this world to reinstate dharma and their commitment to love and devotion.

> "May Lakshmi Devi's blessings shower abundantly over all beings and elevate the quality of our human love to the heights of ecstatic devotional love and elevate our minds to the level of transcendence."

Shakti and Shiva complement each other and are worshipped both separately and together within their cosmic dance of manifestation and emancipation. Shiva without his Shakti is a *shava*, or corpse, in this manifest reality, and at the same time, Shiva is all-pervading within the entirety of cosmic creation.

Shakti as the consort of Shiva is named Sati, the devi of pure truth; she is called Parvati as the mother of Ganesha and Skanda and the daughter of the mountain; she is Durga as the fortress and protective power; and she is Kali as the primal force and controller of time.

Shiva in his many forms is called Mahadeva, the great god; Rudra, the terrible; Nataraja, the cosmic dancer; Shambu, the bestower of auspiciousness; and Pinakin, one who has a bow in his hand.

As a yogini, I feel the power and the blessings of this divine couple in particular in my everyday sadhana. Bringing forth the energy of transformation, these two archetypes, or deities, hold much symbolism, represent sacred wisdom and teachings, and provide spiritual nourishment and guardianship to their devotees.

> "May the mother of the universe, Jagadambe, bless you with her power of creation to increase vitality and awaken love. May the great god, Mahadeva, bless you with the power of discrimination to destroy ignorance and awaken wisdom."

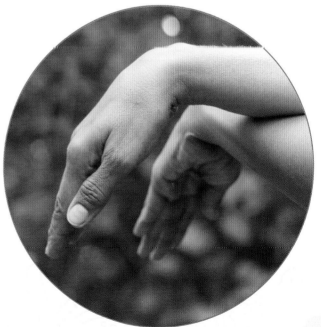

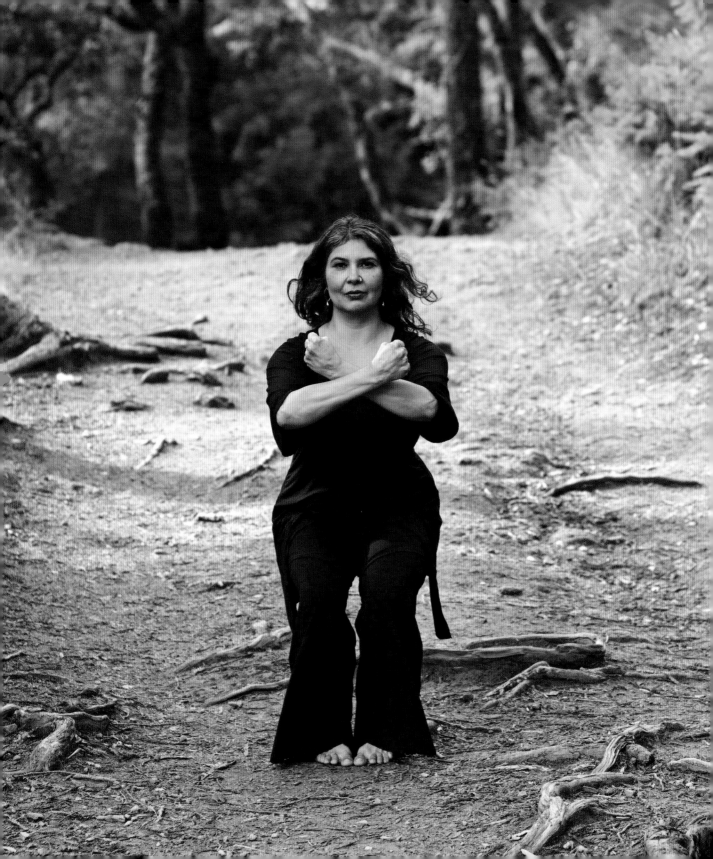

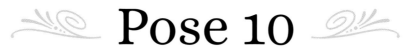

Pose 10

Utkatasana with *musti kavaca mudra*

Mudra

Musti means "strength" and *kavaca* means "shield." Inhale from your abdomen through to your lungs while closing your hands in a fist and gathering the willpower from your navel area into the heart area. Cross your forearms in front of your chest, creating a shield-like mudra, and with the determination to protect and be protected, open your eyes to see clearly what or who is in need of support.

Asana

Bring your feet together, and as you sit back by bending the knees, align your knees with the centers of your feet. Find length in the sides of your body, and move the front ribs in to engage your abdomen. Sit deeper, and feel the work that's happening in your thighs.

Utkatasana is translated as "the fierce pose." Awakening strength and determination, stay firm in your body while holding this pose. Bring your hands to the *musti* shield in front of your heart, relax your shoulders, and imagine a force field of fierce love all around you.

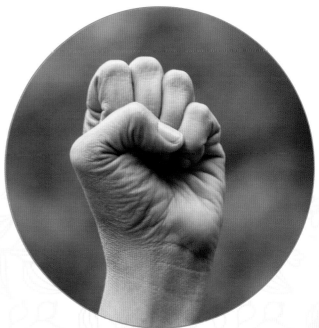

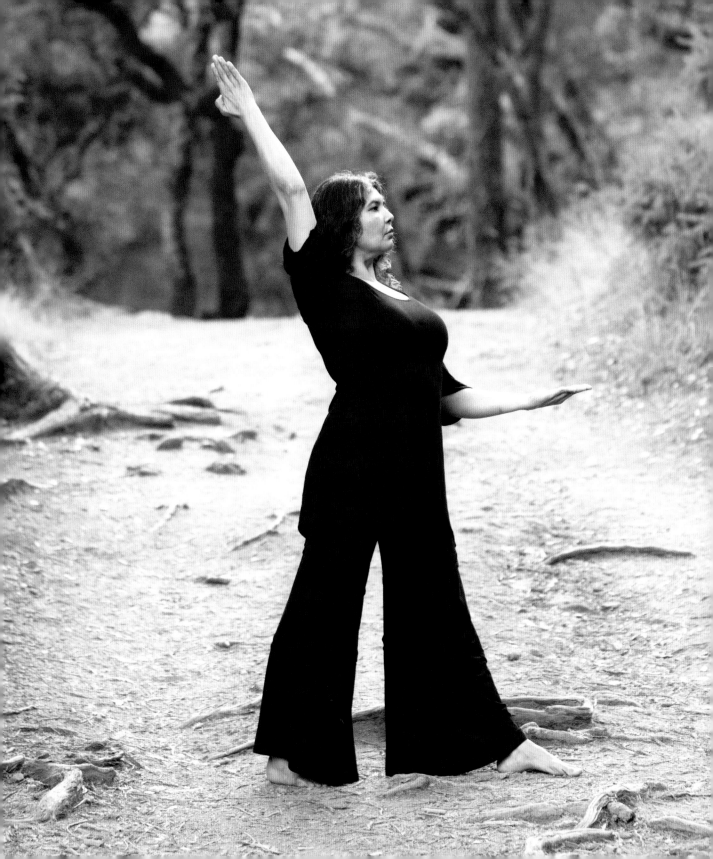

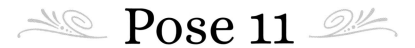

Pose 11

Kali bijasana, rekha pada with *pataka mudra*

"om klim kalikayei namaha"

*"May I come near to your compassionate
shelter, held by your hands of purification,
and become capable of seeing beyond the
veils into the eternal."*

Mudra

In this abhinaya, the *pataka mudra* above the
head shows Kali's sword, and the *pataka mudra* in
the hand by the hips resembles Kali's bowl of blood.
The inner attitude in adopting this mudra is of victory and power. Here, Kali Ma is bringing her strong
medicine of righteousness and justice to the world.
She is the fierce mother who won't allow any evil to
pervade.

Asana

In this Odissi stance, start with your feet parallel and
slightly apart. Step your right foot 2 feet back, and
keep your hips facing forward. Distribute your body
weight between both sides, and stand tall and with
pride by lifting the heart center and the chin slightly
upward. The sense of embodying fearlessness is the
essence of this pose. As you stand tall and firm with
your feet on the ground, be ready to use your sword
of justice if necessary.

This is the pose of Kali standing on top of her
Lord Shiva. In the story of her springing from Mother
Durga's third eye in order to destroy the demon Rak-
tabija, she begins her unstoppable killing. The only
way that she was contained was by surprise, when
she noticed that she was standing on her beloved
Shiva, and just as she's about to kill him, she freezes
and sticks her tongue out in surprise.

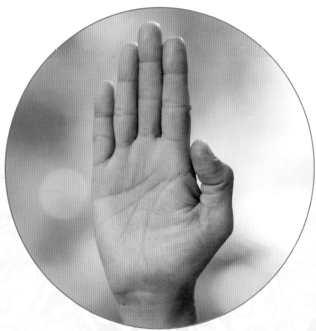

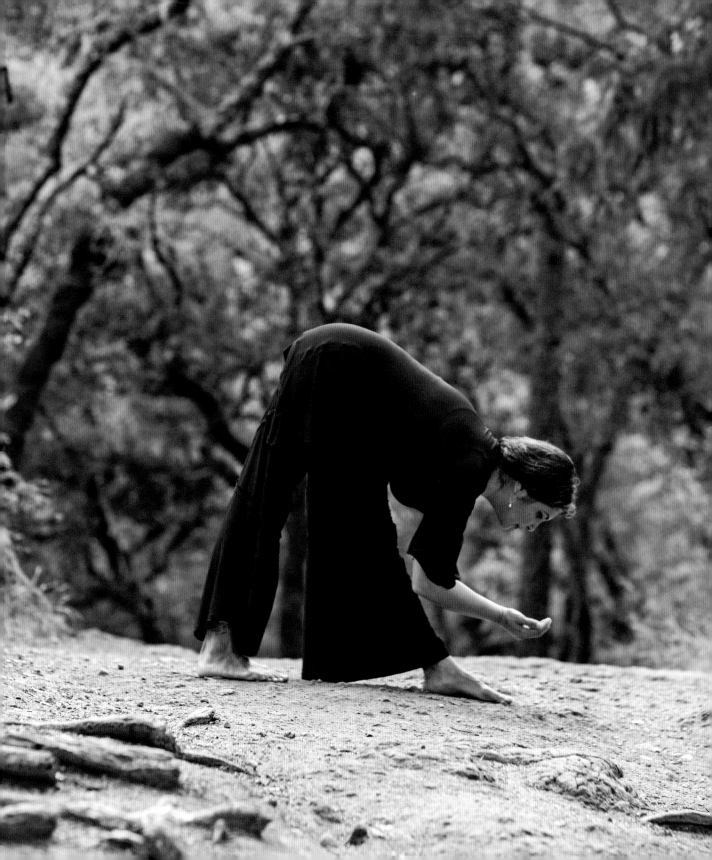

Pose 12

Uttana rekha pada with *pushpaputa mudra*

Mudra

The *pushpaputa* hand gesture represents an offering to be placed at the feet of Mother Kali. Bring your hands together in prayer mudra, and open your palms inward by keeping your fingers together and slightly curved in the shape of an offering bowl. Bring to mind the shadowy parts of yourself that you would like to offer to Kali, knowing that her energy of destruction creates space for the new, and pour your heart into this offering. This mother of mercy is capable of dealing with the most negative forces, and out of kindness, she consumes these forces within her darkness to bring light back into the world.

Asana

Begin the pose by standing with feet parallel and bringing your hands to *pushpaputa mudra*. Bend the knees, and lean forward to step your right foot back at about a 2-foot distance from the left, keeping your right foot aligned with the right hip. Align the right outer heel with the little toe, and fold forward with the front knee, bent at first. Hinge from the hips, and keep your chest open. If it feels right, stretch the left leg, and when you feel balanced, look at your hands while lifting your chin slightly. Take your time to do your own offering and converse with Mother Kali. To come up and out, bend your front knee.

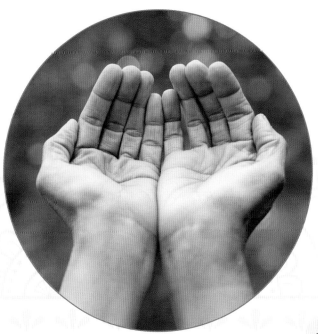

Pose 13

Utkata konasana with hands in *trikona mudra*

Mudra

The triangle mudra, or *trikona*, can be used either with the base of the triangle facing up, as an upside-down triangle, or with the base of the triangle facing down, as a right-side-up triangle. The difference in the symbolism is that the upside-down triangle represents the feminine, and the right-side-up triangle represents the masculine.

For the purpose of this pose, we will have the triangle facing down as we visualize this mudra in a red color, creating the symbol of the fire element in the abdomen area. Unite the tips of the thumbs, and unite the tips of the index fingers, keeping the rest of the fingers together and the palms flat, creating the shape of an equilateral triangle with your hands.

Asana

Stand tall and separate your feet about 3 feet apart. Point your toes out, and while bending the knees, keep the back of your body aligned. Find a connection to the central line along your spine, or *shushumna*, and push the tailbone to the earth while lifting the crown of the head up to the sky. Relax your shoulders, and bring your hands in *trikona mudra* to the navel area. Call upon the power of the earth and the power of fire. As you place your feet on the earth, awaken the inner fire in your belly and in your *ajna* chakra, or third eye. Bring in your mind's eye one of your goals, and visualize that you are strong and capable of bringing this goal to fruition with sharp focus and dedication.

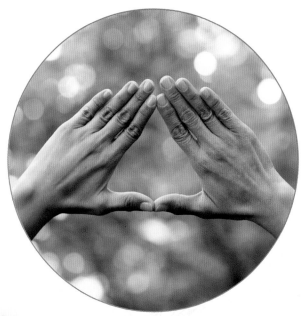

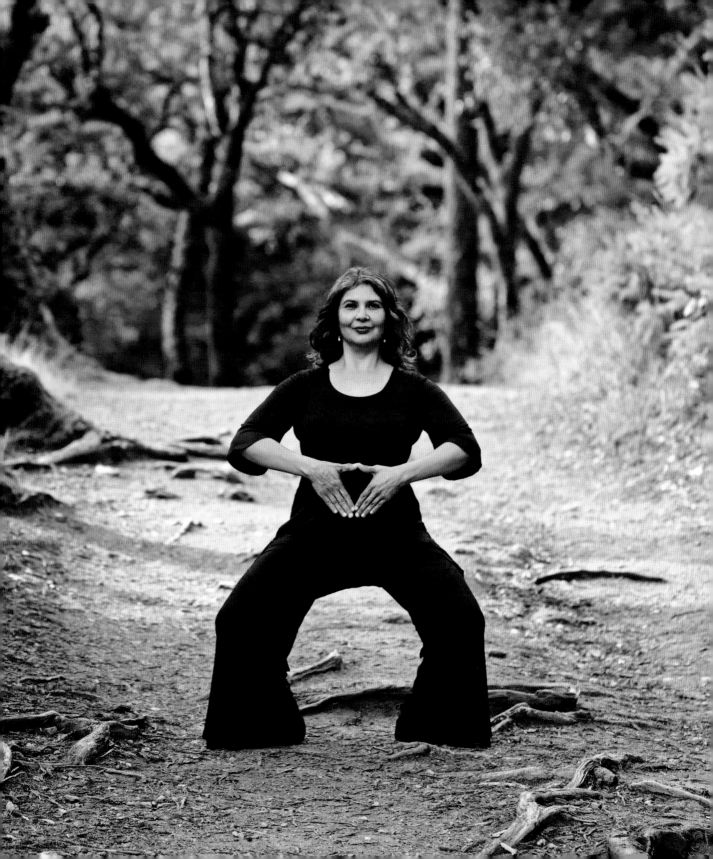

Pose 14

Virabhadrasana one with *shanka mudra*

Mudra

The blowing of the conch announces new beginnings and victory. The conch shell is one of Durga's attributes, and she uses it as a weapon of protection. The sound of the conch will destroy anything that has not come into the world of manifestation yet. It will purify and destroy the lower vibrational frequencies of impure thoughts or inferior beings.

Open your left palm, and stretch your left thumb up, with the four fingers of your right hand enveloping the left thumb. Touch the right thumb to the left index finger while placing the side of the left index finger at the second phalanges of the four fingers on the right hand. Now, place the rest of the four fingers of the left hand on the back of the right hand, until the left little finger touches the knuckles of the right hand.

Asana

In this asana, we are telling the story of Durga using her weapon *shanka*, or conch shell, to annihilate the evil that is pervading her grounds. In "warrioress" one, start with your feet together, and get your shell ready in your hands. Step your left foot back, about 3 feet apart, and align heel to heel. The front foot remains pointing forward and the right knee pointing toward the middle toe, while the back foot turns to a 45-degree angle and the outer edge of the left foot presses down on the floor. Your torso is facing the right leg as best you can. Lift the side body while lifting your hands in *shanka mudra* to your mouth, and keep your shoulders down while opening your elbows away from the central line.

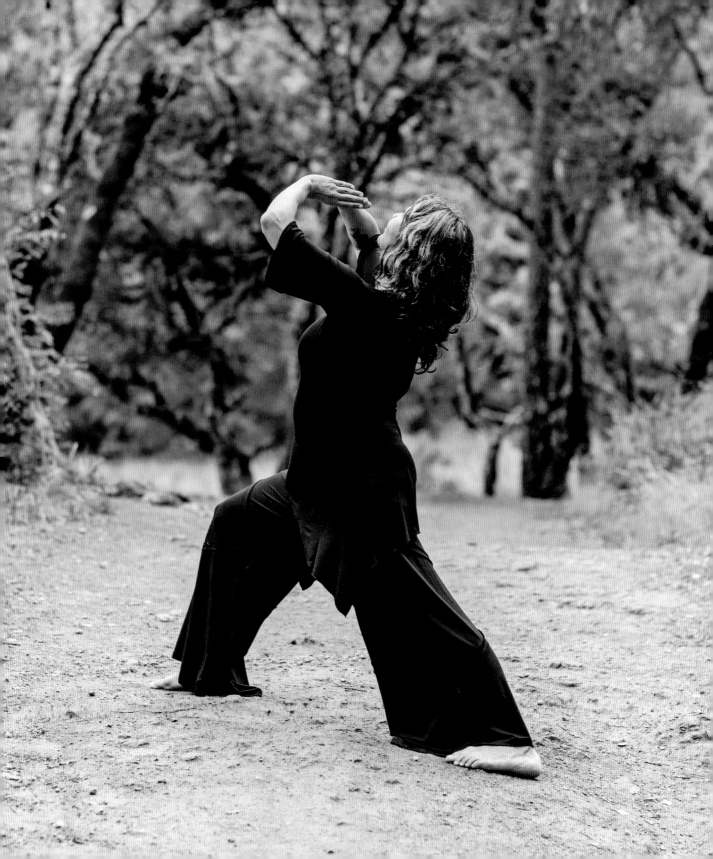

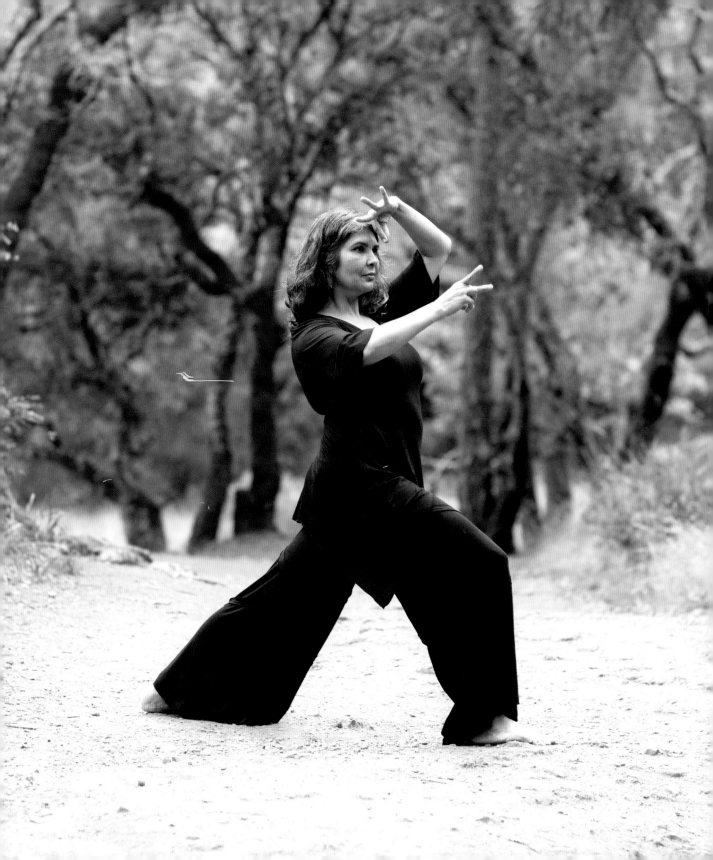

Pose 15

Virabhadrasana one with one hand in *hamsasya mudra* and one hand in *kartarimukha mudra*

Mudras

For *hamsasya*, bring the left thumb to touch the left index finger, and open all the other fingers out. Place this hand between the eyebrows with the index finger and thumb facing down, making the shape of an eye, and the other fingers opening like eyelashes.

For *kartarimukha*, start with peace fingers, stretching right index and middle fingers up while connecting the thumb to the ring and little fingers. As you motion your hands from your third eye, *hamsasya*, forward, open in *kartarimukha*, like the opening of a scissor, showing the fire of the third eye springing forth.

Asana

Start in warrioress one, with the front right knee pointing toward the front right foot and the torso facing forward, while the back left leg is firm and the left inner thigh is moving backward and up. You can combine breath and movement, with the in breath stretching the right leg and bring the *kartarimukha* hand closer to the *hamsasya* hand. With the out breath, bend the front leg and move your fire flame from the third eye forward, clearing whatever is necessary for you to open the path ahead, while you meditate on empowerment by the Divine Mother's clear vision.

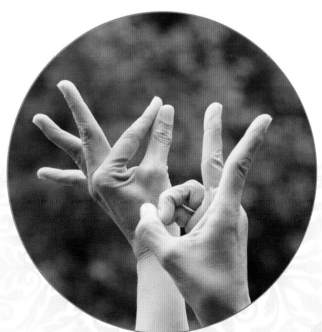

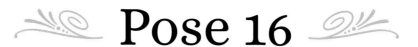

Pose 16

Patadgraha mudra, begging bowl or feeding bowl hand gesture

I normally use this mudra to ask for divine alms in the form of insight and guidance. Here, I chose this mudra to approach Annapurna Devi, who, in her benevolent role of feeding all beings, is completely indiscriminate. Her food grows in her earthly lap for all beings to enjoy her bounty. The story says that even Shiva, the lord of the universe whose beloved is Parvati herself, approaches with his begging bowl, to ask Mother Parvati as Annapurna for material and spiritual nourishment. *Anna* means "food" or "nourishment," and *purna* means "fullness." Anna-purna, therefore, is one of the aspects of the Divine Mother, and her form brings to our attention the need to nourish and honor this physical body of ours, or *anna-maya-kosha.*

Ganesha is never fully satisfied with any food that is not provided by his mother, Parvati (Anna-purna). Her offerings nourish his body, heart, and soul. There is an endearing story where Ganesha gets invited by Kubera, the god of all wealth, to a lunch where Kubera wants to show off his wealth to Ganesha. Ganesha starts eating all of the fanciest dishes and desserts from Kubera's kitchen but comments that he simply does not get satisfied. Time passes, and Kubera has nothing else to serve, so Ganesha starts to eat all of the silverware, the plates, the tables, and just as Ganesha is about to eat the entire palace, Kubera calls Mother Parvati and asks her for any food prepared by her hand to offer Ganesha. A simple bowl of porridge is brought, and after eating his mother's food, Ganesha voices a big sigh of satisfaction and leaves Kubera's home feeling pleased.

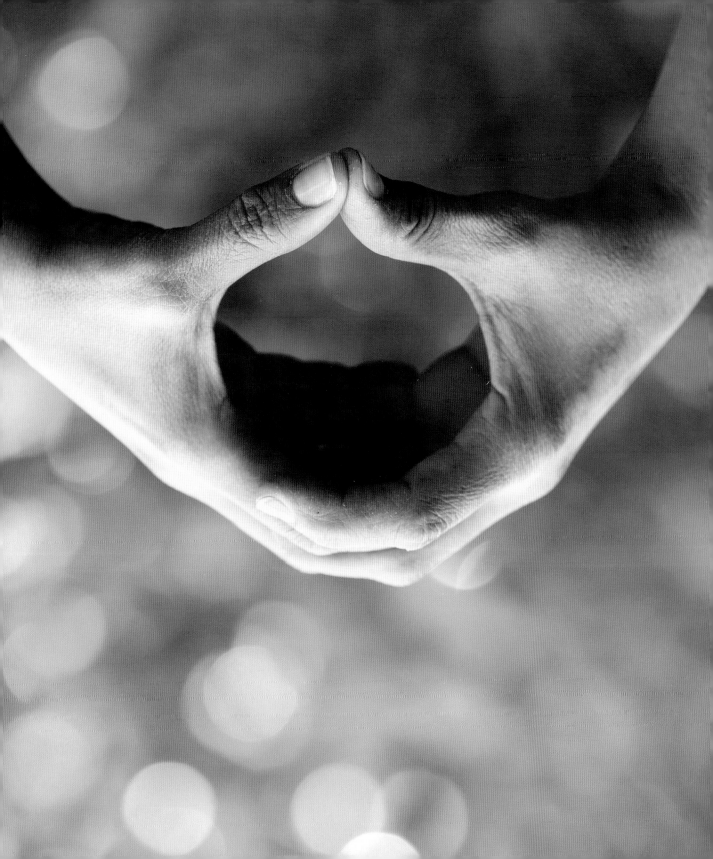

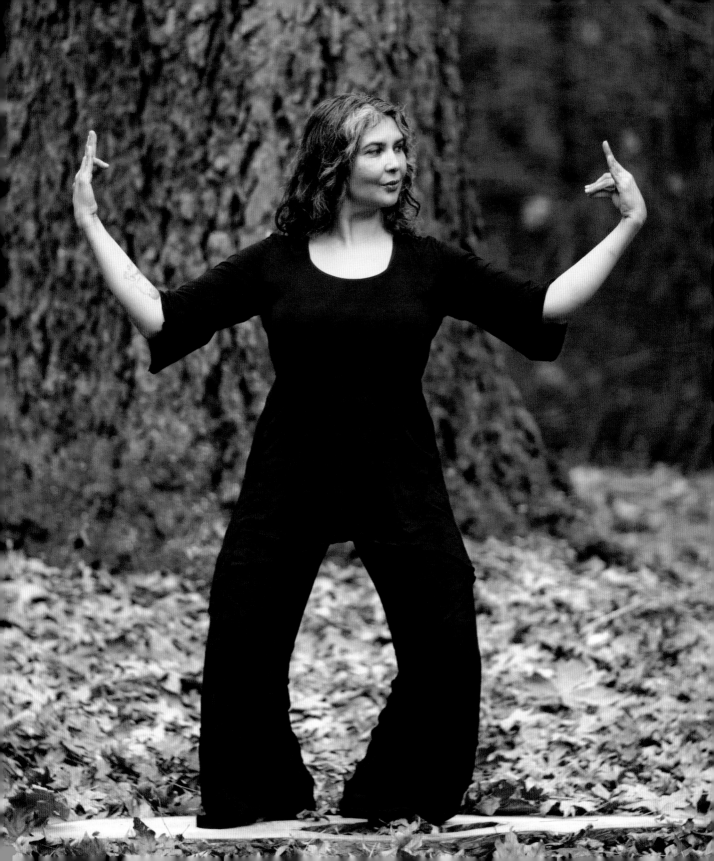

Pose 17

Shiva bijasana, biparitamukha pada with right hand
in *mrgasirsa mudra* and left hand in *tripataka mudra*

Mudras

Mrgasirsa mudra symbolizes the head of a deer. Connect the thumb to the middle and ring fingers while lifting the index and little fingers upward. This is a poetic mudra, and here it is used for Shiva to describe Shiva as Pashupati, or the protector of the animals.

Tripataka is associated to many different male gods, and in some cases, it describes a crown, though this hand gesture can also signify an arrow or a thunderbolt.

From a flat palm, *pataka*, bend the first phalange of your ring finger.

Asana

With your feet together or slightly apart, point your toes and knees out and bend the knees while aligning the kneecaps over the third toe. Sit as deep as you can, or as deep as feels comfortable. Start in alignment with the central line of the body, then take a moment to turn your head to the right and to the left.

Legend in Nepal has it that Shiva as Pashupati Nath, the lord of the animals, lived as a deer by the banks of the river Bagmati, where later a temple dedicated to him was established. Shiva is well known to be the friend of all, the protector of the downtrodden, the benefactor of the lost spirits, the night watcher over our dreams, and the ruler of time.

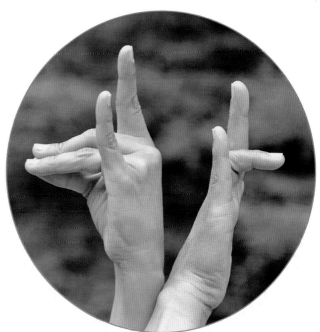

Pose 18

Shiva Nataraja bijasana one, kunchita pada with right hand in *abhaya mudra* and left hand in *dola hasta mudra*

Mudras

Abhaya, with right palm facing forward and fingers up, offering protection.

Dola, with left back of the hand facing out and the fingers pointing down, offering refuge.

Asana

In this Odissi stance, you will be working on balance and foundation while embodying Shiva's merciful pose of tandava dance, where while dancing he offers protection and shelter to his devotees.

Start with your feet together, and open the tops of your feet out. As you bend the knees, activate your legs and define your balance by focusing on the central line of the body and keeping the back of the body aligned. Now transfer the weight to the sole of the right foot while placing the balls of the left toes in front of the arch of the right foot. Keep the knees bent and pointing sideways. Add the mudras, and move the hands over to the right side of the body. With *bhava* and introspection, embody Shiva's force and his message: "Fear not, you are safe under my shelter."

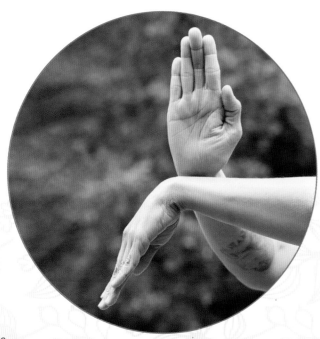

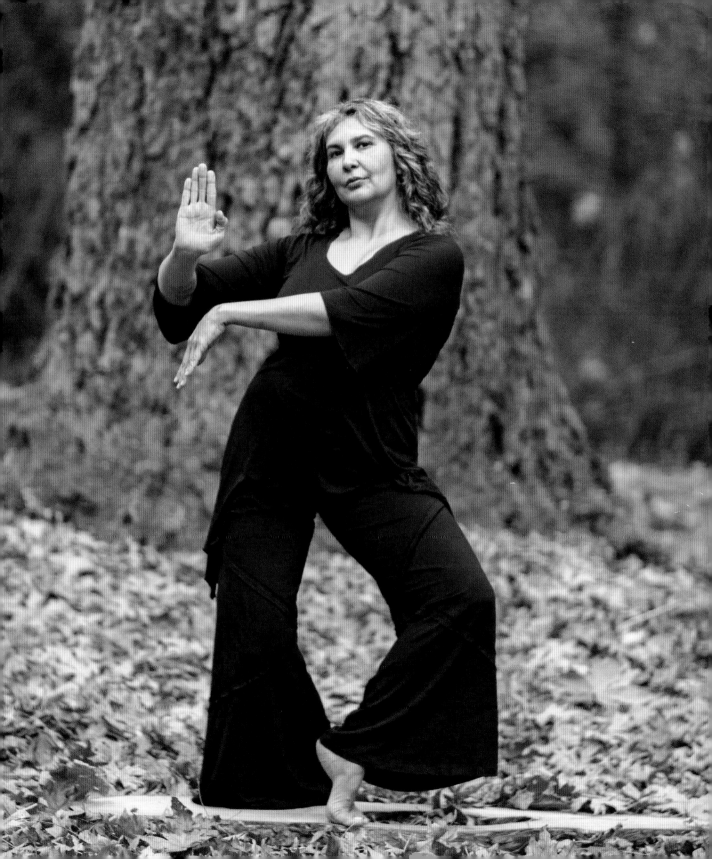

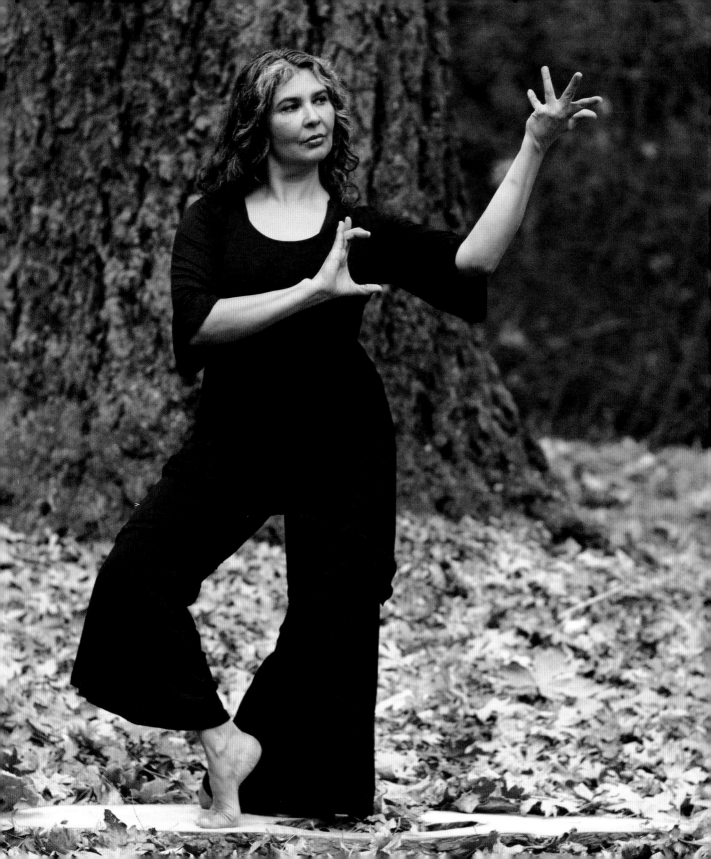

Pose 19

Shiva Nataraja bijasana two, kunchita pada with left hand in *alapadma mudra* and right hand in *damaru mudra*

Mudras

Alapadma: Begin with your left palm flat facing upward, and separate your thumb from the base of the index finger while pointing the index finger. Move your middle finger higher than the index finger, the ring finger higher than the middle finger, and the pinkie higher than the ring finger, creating a shape of the rays of the sun with your hand. This mudra in this pose symbolizes Shiva's fire of destruction.

Damaru: Begin with your right hand in *pataka*, and imagine you are holding a small two-headed drum called *damaru*. With your thumb, hold its base, and with your middle and ring fingers, hold its top, with the index and little fingers pointing up. In this pose, this hand gesture represents the sound of creation.

Asana

In this Odissi pose, the iconography of Shiva destroys with the fire of purification that which is unreal and ephemeral. At the same time, he creates with the sound of his drum that which is real and eternal.

Start with your feet together, and open the tops of your feet out to bend the knees while aligning the knees over the feet. Now transfer the weight to the sole of the left foot while placing the balls of the right toes in front of the arch of the left foot. Add the mudras, the mood, and the intention to make peace with the ever-changing currents of life.

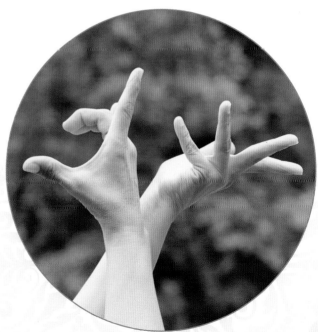

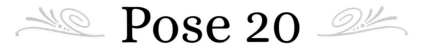

Pose 20

Vishnu and Jagannath mudras

"jagannath swami nayana patha gami bhavatu me"

"May Lord Jagannath be the object of my vision."

When holding *tripataka mudra* in both hands, you will be depicting Lord Vishnu in his universal form, the sustainer of the universe, as well as in his form as Jagannath, the bringer of joy and delight. The mood of *maha-bhava*, supreme sentiment and enraptured bliss, is encapsulated in Sri Jagannath's big loving eyes, in his endearing smile, and in his transcendental form.

The story says that Sri Krishna assumed the form of Jagannath, along with his brother Balarama and his sister Subhadra, when they got enchanted by listening to the pastimes and love stories of the *gopis* of Vrindavan. The mood of nectar was so intense that these three deities froze and withdrew their senses. At that time, Narada Muni, the celestial musician, entered the space where they were and witnessed this special form of the Lord. Dancing with his arms up in the air, Narada said, "I have seen it! I have seen it! And I beg you to keep this form in order to delight your devotees!" So, to fulfill Narada's desire, Krishna remained in Puri as Lord Jagannath.

Other mudras for Sri Vishnu are the *shanka* or conch shell, the *chakra* or discus, the *gada* or mace, and the *padma* or lotus.

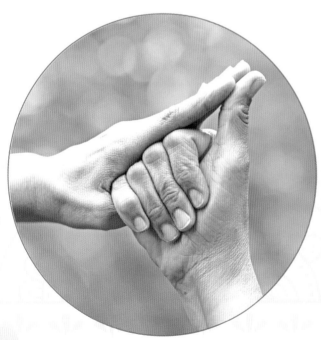

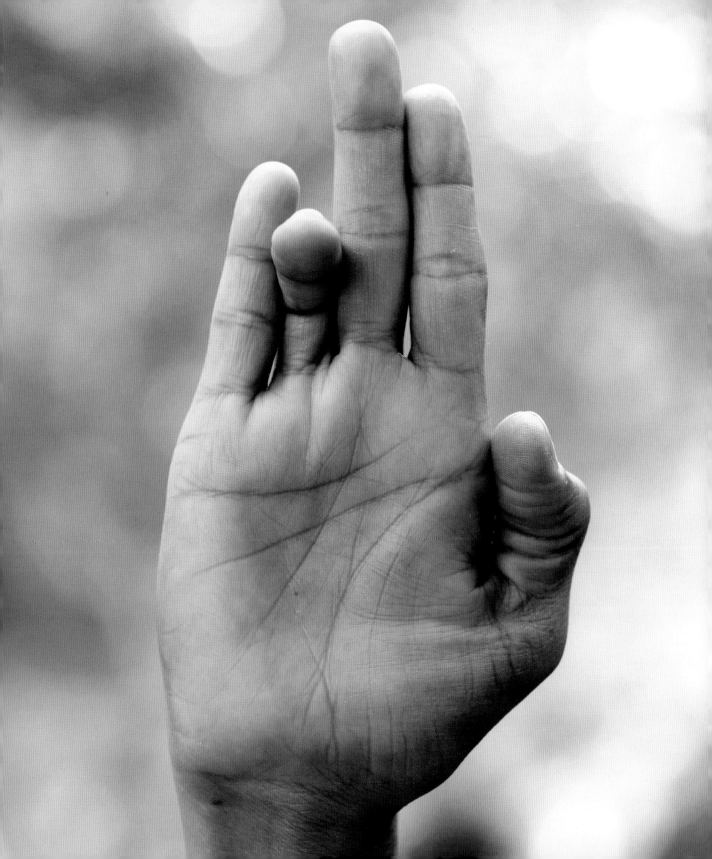

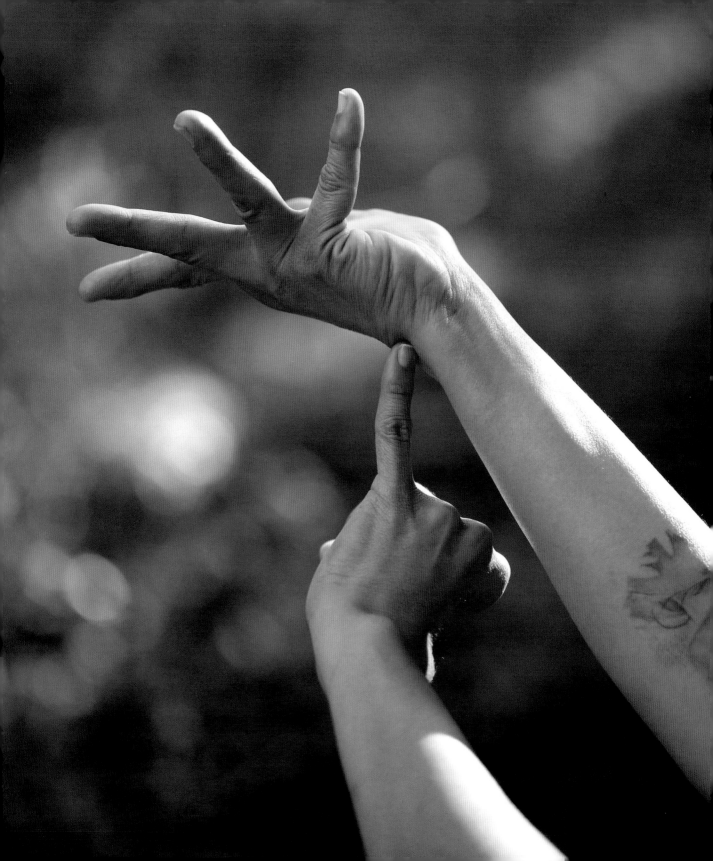

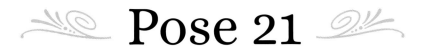

Pose 21

Lakshmi and *Bhumi Devi mudras*

When uniting *bana mudra* (little finger pointing out) to an *alapadma mudra* in the way shown in this photo, you can envision the upward journey of a lotus flower from the muddy waters to the sky. I called this the *Kamala mudra.*

The symbol of the lotus is depicting Lakshmi as Kamala Devi, she who is of the lotus, and in this aspect, she reveals her beauty and perfection to us. Kamala Devi also shows us that the path from darkness to light is a trajectory of bringing forth her auspiciousness.

Mother Lakshmi is also known as Mother Earth or Bhumi Devi. This second mudra, I call *gola mudra,*

gola meaning "geode," "globe," or another sphere-like thing. I associate this hand gesture to Mother Earth with one of her many gifts to us because all of the precious stones can be considered part of her womb. Containing the power and the richness of Bhumi Devi, this unbroken geode is a sacred cave to access her mysteries and her beauty.

Thinking also of *gola mudra* as representing the globe, we hold this hand gesture in our hands as we understand that the power to preserve and sustain this planet is within our reach and within each of our positive actions.

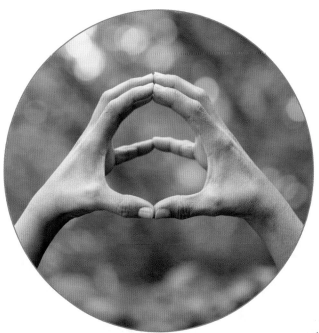

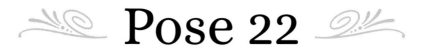

Pose 22

Samputa mudra

Mudra

This mudra refers to a secret, or a message. Make a bowl with your hands and place the palm of the right hand on top of the left palm, holding your treasure between your palms.

In this abhinaya, we are referring to Lord Hanuman carrying a message from Rama to Sita during her imprisonment by Ravana.

Ramayana retold by Jai Uttal

Many eons ago, or perhaps right now, in a parallel universe, the material plane of existence was slowly but surely shattering. All the universes, all the planets, and all the realms were being destroyed by the demon king Ravana and his many minions. Evil was triumphing over dharma.

In desperation, the gods went to see Lord Vishnu—the indwelling spirit, Hari, the beloved, the Alpha and Omega—and begged him to help. From his heavenly repose in Vaikuntha, he looked down and saw the suffering of all beings and said, "Yes, I will descend to Earth in a material form as Rama, son of King Dasharatha of Ayodhya." Vishnu's eternal consort, Maha Lakshmi, said, "If you're going, so am I! I will take birth as Sita, in the family of King Janaka, the wise."

So they were born as "humans": Rama of blue skin with his three brothers, Lakshmana, Bharata, and Satrughna, and, in a neighboring kingdom, Sita, the daughter of the earth. Lord Shiva, from his heavenly abode on Mount Kailash, also wanted to come and help his beloved Hari, so he assumed the diminutive form of an all-powerful, all-knowing monkey named Hanuman.

As Rama and his brothers grew up, the day for Rama's coronation arrived. But, by a cruel twist of fate and destiny, Rama, Sita, and Lakshmana were exiled to the forest for fourteen years. During this period of exile, they lived quite happily until the demon king Ravana, in his lust for power, abducted Sita. Rama subsequently fell apart in the anguish of separation. It was at this point that Hanuman made his appearance and offered his help to Rama.

Hanuman immediately recognized the blue-skinned forest dweller as the Supreme Being and fell to the ground, overcome with emotion. So an alliance was formed between Rama, Lakshmana, Hanuman, and all of the creatures of the natural world, particularly the monkeys and the bears. They found Sita imprisoned in Lanka in the palace of Ravana, and a huge war ensued to free the goddess. During this conflict, Hanuman proved to be the greatest of devotees and the greatest of warriors.

Finally, Rama defeated Ravana and was reunited with Sita. Rama, Sita, Lakshmana, Hanuman, and the vast armies flew in an aerial chariot back to Ayodhya, where they were greeted with hundreds of thousands of lamps lighting their way, both from Heaven and from Earth. This moment is celebrated in India and throughout the world as Diwali, the festival of lights.

Rama was coronated, and with Sita by his side, he ruled the world for a hundred thousand years in what is called the golden age of harmony, after which they ascended back to the heavens.

This is, of course, an abbreviated version of one of the most amazing stories ever told. Whether one sees it as a metaphor, a fairy tale, a spiritual story, or pure history does not matter; the journey of Rama is filled with so much emotion, both human and divine, along with such transcendence that it cannot help but transform the listener's inner world. Such is the power and beauty of Bhakti.

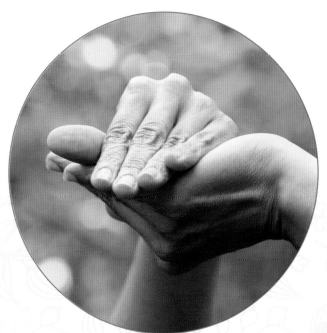

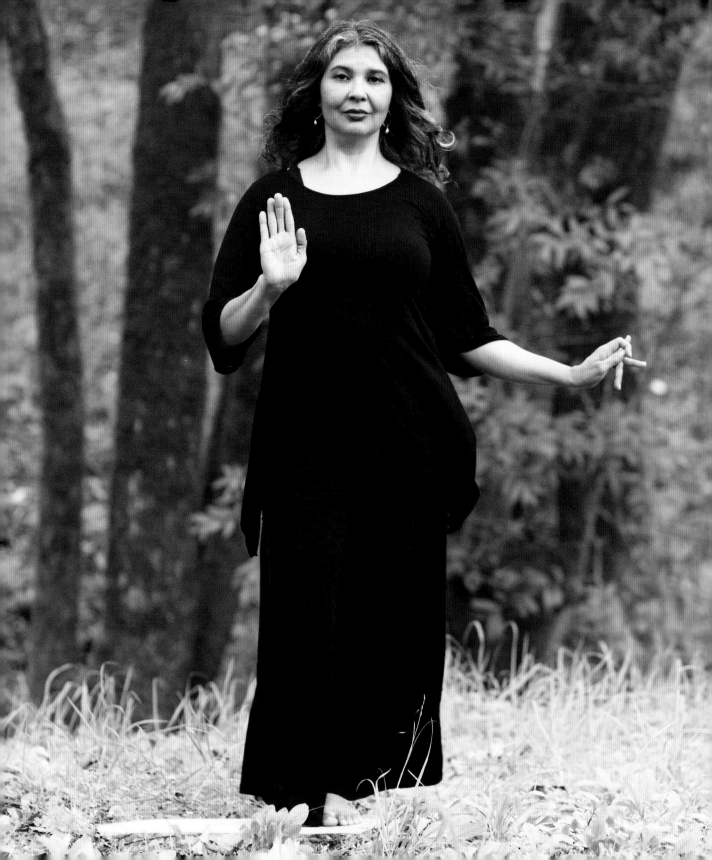

Pose 23

Sita bijasana, abhanga pada with right hand in *ardhachandra* as *abhaya mudra* and left hand in *katakamukha mudra*

Mudras

Katakamukha mudra, holding a lotus flower. Connect your left index finger with the top of the left thumb, while the left middle finger points to the palm and the ring and pinkie fingers are pointing away from the palm.

Abhaya mudra, offering protection and granting a blessing. Hold the right palm facing forward while shining the light forth from the heart.

Asana

Abhanga is a very common stance for the Devi. In this pose, Sita Devi is depicted in this uneven pose showering her blessings upon us. From a standing pose, simply bend your right knee while holding the mudras and gazing forward toward creation or anyone you wish to bring unconditional love to.

Mother Sita comes empowering us with the qualities of loyalty, simplicity, patience, and endurance. Her faithfulness and dedication to her beloved Rama brings to us the teaching of strength of refuge. When in despair, never doubt that your Lord will come to the rescue.

Sita was abducted by the evil demon Ravana, and through the most horrifying situations, she always kept her single-pointed mind on her savior, Rama, and she never compromised her loyalty.

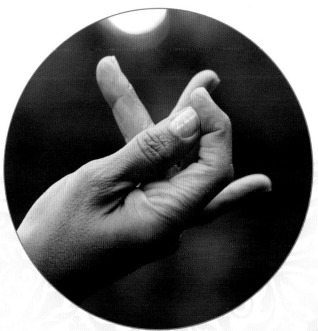

Pose 24

Rama bijasana, dhanu pada with hands in *katakamukha two mudra*

Mudra

Katakamukha in this pose is used to show Rama holding his bow in the right hand and an arrow on the left hand. Start with your thumb up, and bring the pad of your index finger to touch the top of the thumb. Now stretch the middle finger down toward the palm and point the ring and little fingers slightly up.

Asana

Simply stand tall on both feet and, after ensuring you feel firm, transfer your body weight to your left foot while crossing the right foot in front of the left. Open the right knee out, and place the balls of the right toes on the ground across the left side of the body.

Ramachandra, as one of the avatars of Lord Vishnu, brought to us humans the example of morality and virtue. To fulfill his mission on the earth, he incarnated as the son of Dasharatha in the city of Ayodhya. In order to observe his father's honor, he was exiled from his kingdom for fourteen years. Along with his beloved wife Sita and his dearest brother Lakshman, Rama wandered the forest as a mendicant, without any privilege, out of his undeterred sense of duty. The bow and arrow is his signature weapon and one of his only possessions.

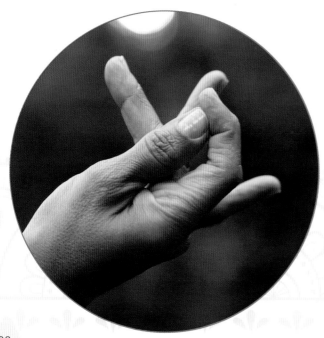

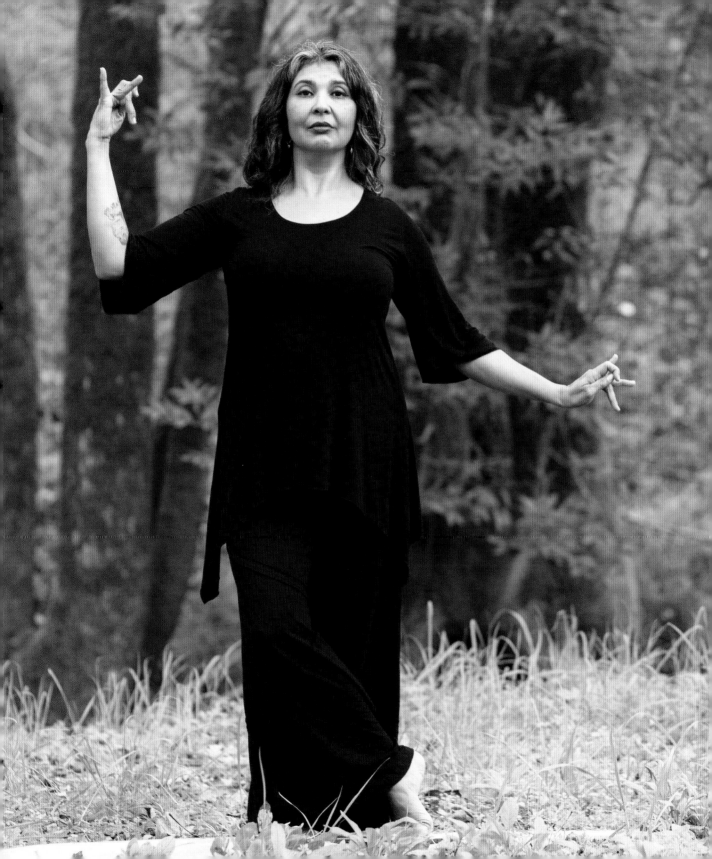

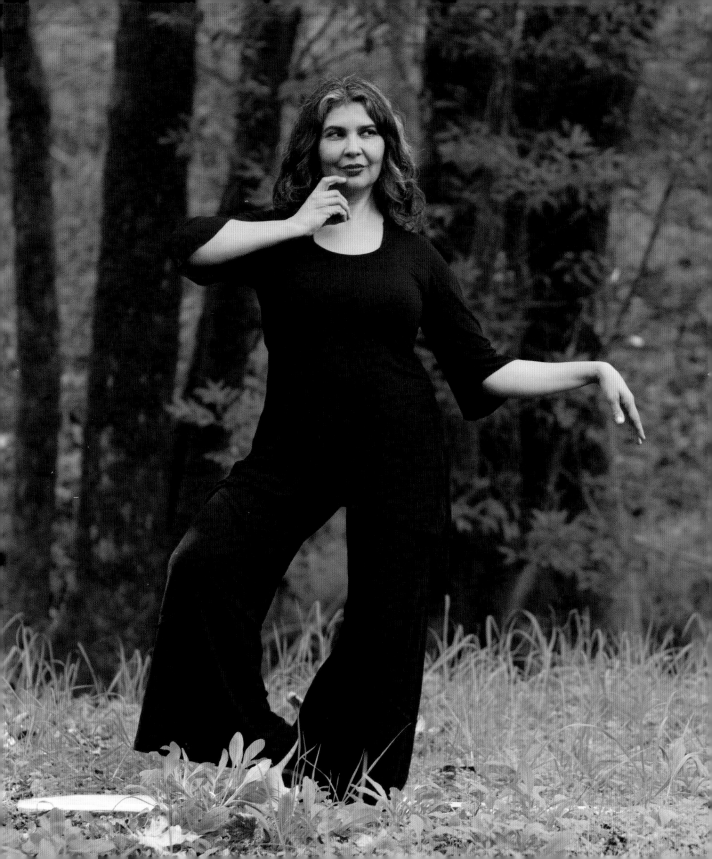

Pose 25

Radha bijasana one, kunchita pada with right hand in *tamrachuda mudra* and left hand in *dola hasta mudra*

Mudras

For *tamrachuda mudra* in the right hand, connect the thumb to the little, ring, and middle fingers, and stretch your index finger like the tip of a hook, placing it by the corner of the mouth.

For *dola hasta mudra*, relax the fingers of your left hand slightly pointing down to the earth while bending by the wrist and feeling the lightness of your arms and fingers.

Asana

In this pose, Sri Radharani is walking through the forest looking with longing eyes for Sri Krishna, her beloved. She walks with her hips swinging from side to side, and she glances between the leaves of the thick forest looking for him, trying to see him. She senses his presence and hears the sound of his flute, but she cannot see him, and her mood of longing becomes contagious, engaging nature and creation all around her.

Turn the toes out as you bend the knees. Place the right toes on the earth in front of the arch of left foot, and find your balance, keeping your center in alignment with the central line of the spine. Let your hips slightly sway to the left, and place your right hand in *tamrachuda* by the chin and your left hand in *dola* by your hip.

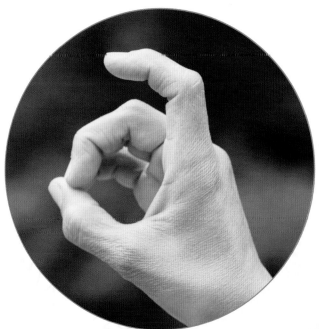

Pose 26

Radha bijasana two, kunchita pada with left hand in *katakamukha two mudra* and right hand in *dola hasta mudra*

Mudras

We have used the *katakamukha mudra* many times previously, but here it describes Radha covering her beautiful face with the top part of her sari while trying to hide from Krishna.

Dola hasta on the right hand is showing the beauty of Radha's gracefulness.

Asana

In this pose, Sri Radha finds her beloved Krishna in the midst of a sweet *kunja*, or grove, in the forest. Radha becomes aware of Krishna's loving glimpses and becomes shy, hiding her moonlike face behind her sari. The love game begins. The play of desiring and pushing away, looking for and hiding from, coming together and separating is the nectar of Radha and Krishna's teachings to us, Radha symbolizing the lover and Krishna the beloved.

Turn the toes and knees out and bend the knees. Place the balls of the left toes on the ground in front of the arch of right foot. Sit deeply and sway your hips a little to the right. The torso will naturally move to the left. While you look slightly down, use your left hand in *katakamukha two* to cover your face a little. The right hand rests in *dola hasta* by the hips.

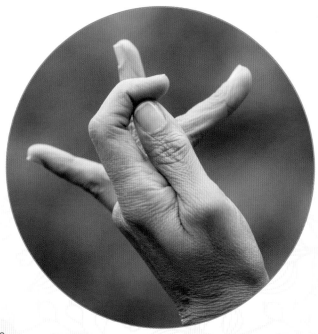

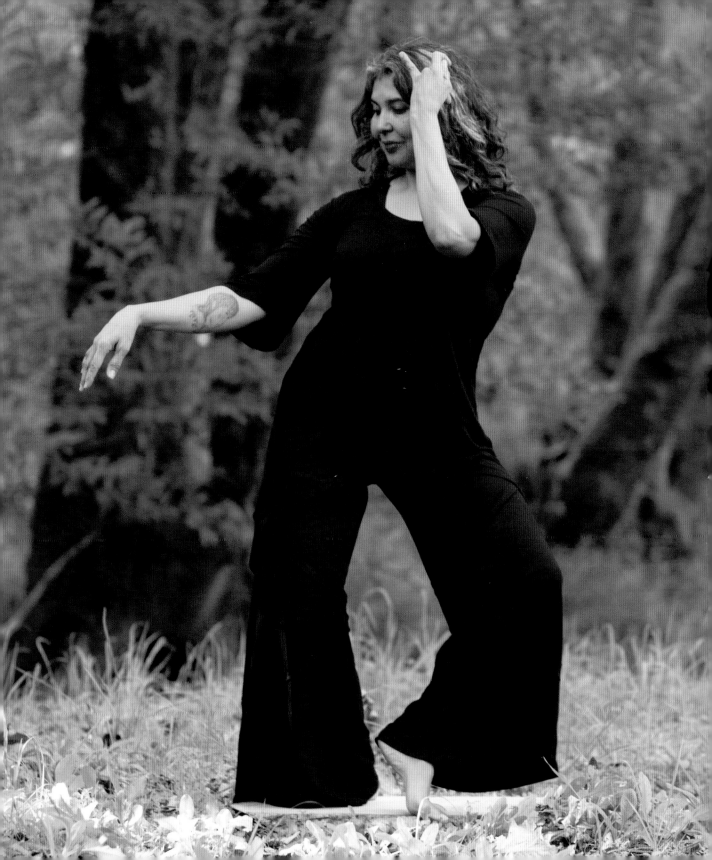

Pose 27

Krishna bijasana one, dhanu pada with
two hands in *mrgasirsa mudra*

Mudra

In the Odissi style of dance, we hold Krishna's flute
with two hands in *mrgasirsa*. In this style, *mrgasirsa*
is when you connect the thumb with the middle
and ring fingers keeping the index and little fingers straight up. In other styles of dance, *mrgasirsa*
is *simhamukha*, and the little finger and thumb are
up, while the index, middle, and ring fingers are held
straight and bent by the knuckles.

While adopting either version of this mudra,
imagine holding a bamboo flute in the space
between the palms.

Asana

From standing pose, open your right foot to the right,
and cross the right foot over to the left while lifting
the right heel and pointing the right knee to the right.
Move your hands over to the right side of the body by
the mouth as you tilt your head just a little bit over
the left shoulder. Now add the mudra to this pose.

Krishna is all-attractive, and when he plays his
flute, we are lured into his realm. The reward of being
in his presence is the awakening of love in all of its
colors and moods. Krishna rekindles the spark of pas-
sion for a life of devotion in the hearts of those that
have lost it, and Krishna quenches the burning fires
of desire of his loving devotees by attending to each
one individually and most intimately.

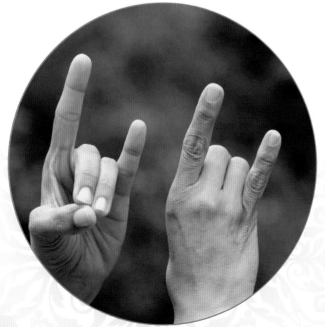

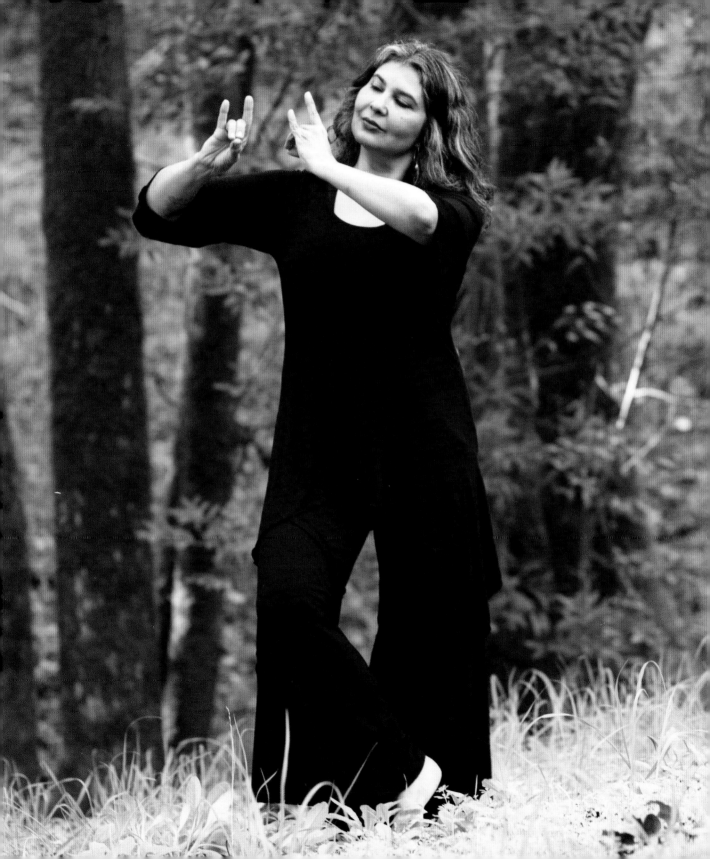

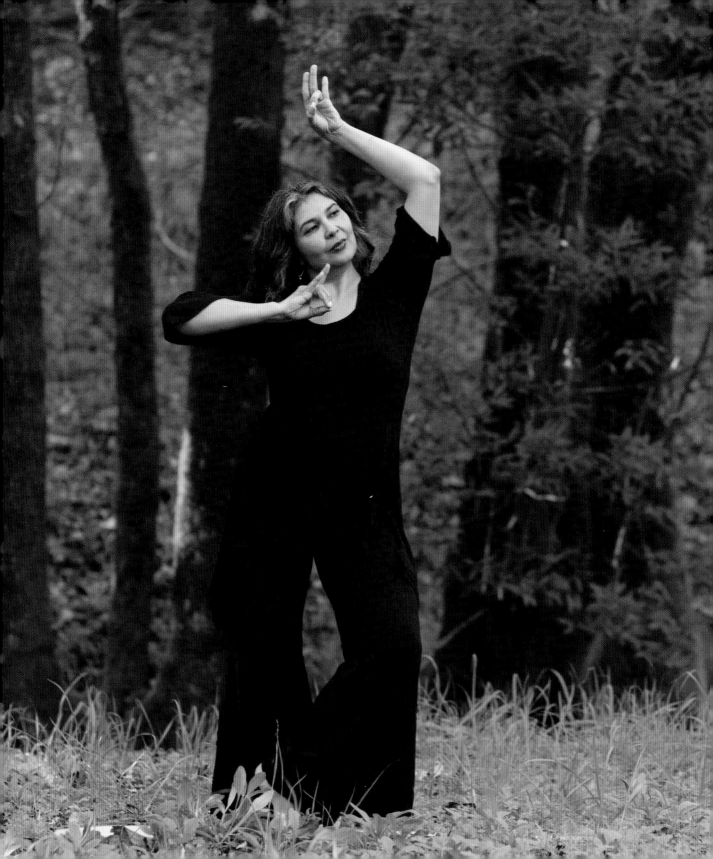

Pose 28

Krishna bijasana two, dhanu pada with left hand in *mayura mudra* and right hand in *mrgasirsa mudra*

Mudras

Mayura mudra is used here as the peacock feather that decorates Krishna's crown. Open your left palm flat, bend the ring finger and thumb, and bring them to touch at the center of your left palm.

Mrgasirsa in the right hand is placed by the lips and represents the flute. Connect the middle and ring fingers to the thumb while lifting the index and little fingers.

Asana

Stand tall and open your left foot out while crossing the left leg in front of the right leg. You could micro-bend your right knee as you place the balls of the left toes over on the right side of the body. Tilt your head to the right, and place your right hand by the chin or mouth, just how you would hold a flute. Place your left hand above the crown of your head like the peacock feather of Krishna.

Krishna's playfulness and multifaceted ways of loving are symbolically represented in how he uses his peacock feather. With it, he teases his lovers with all the colors found around the eye of the feather. Krishna, the most skilled enchanter, awakens all the senses of his devotees and prepares them to experience ultimate bliss.

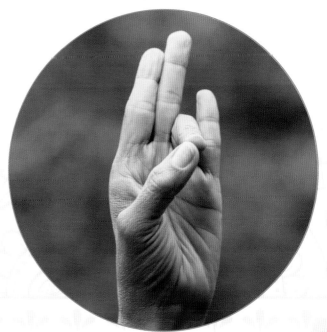

Pose 29

Narayanasana with *nagabandha mudra* as *sesha*

Mudra

Nagabandha mudra here depicts the hood of the five-headed king of the serpents, Nagaraja or Adishesha. *Sesha* is Lord Vishnu's couch, and while Vishnu as Lord Narayana rests his body, his beloved Lakshmi massages his feet.

Bring your thumbs to cross while lifting your arms above your head and curving your hands like the shape of a snake hood. The fingers will be together, and the elbows will bend to accommodate Lord Vishnu's head like a pillow while providing shelter.

This protector snake always follows Vishnu and Lakshmi. He came to this earthly plane as Balarama with Krishna, as Lakshmana with Rama, and as the snake that provided shelter for Buddha closer to the moment of his full enlightenment.

Asana

This is a balance position. Stand tall and place your hands in *nagabandha mudra* over your head. Balancing on your left foot, begin to slide your right foot forward while reclining back in your imaginary couch. Ensure your chin continues to touch your chest, and avoid dropping the head back. The arms are like a pillow for your head, your heart center raises, and you come down with your back parallel to the earth while lifting your right leg up higher. For a more advanced pose, position the entire torso and right leg parallel to the ground, like a reverse warrioress one.

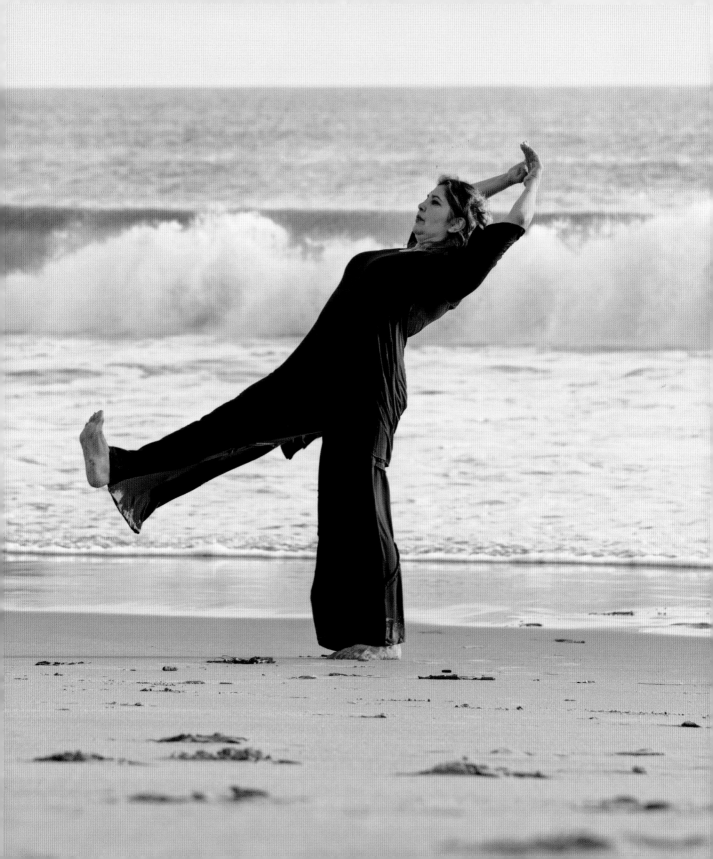

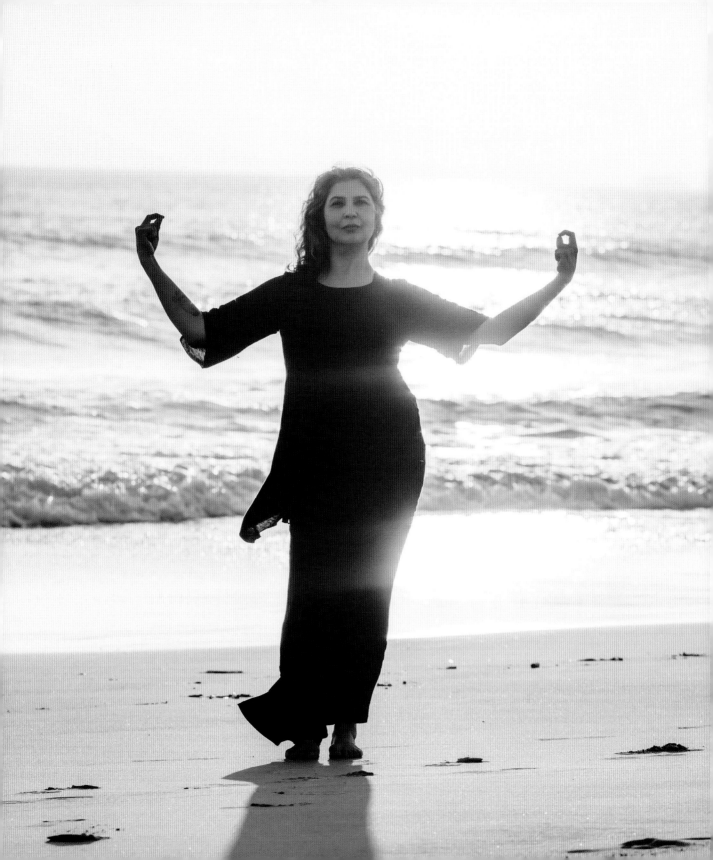

Pose 30

Lakshmi bijasana, abhanga pada with two hands in *kapittha mudra*

"om shrim lakshmiyei namaha"

"May I float on your bountiful nourishing body, held by your hands of love, and become capable of seeing your beauty."

Mudra

Kapittha literally translates as "elephant-apple." In the art of Viniyoga, *kapittha* has many different uses: It can be used to play the cymbals, to milk a cow, as an incense or light offering, to show the crown of the head, and so on. This mudra is often used to denote the goddess Lakshmi as she holds the stems of two lotus flowers by her shoulders and allows the universe to shine with her golden beauty.

Put your thumbs up with the index fingers touching the top of the thumbs. As you bring your hands to shoulder level, move the backs of your hands out and bend the wrists.

Asana

Devi Lakshmi stands in *abhanga*, or an uneven standing position, rising from the ocean of plentifulness. She is the mother of abundance, and her gifts to us, her children, are many. We just need to open our eyes and hearts to see how much we have and how much materially and spiritually she has given us.

Alternatively, for this pose, you may also sit down in *padmasana* or *ardha padmasana*, lotus or half-lotus meditation pose, and perform her other two mudras, *abhaya* and *varada*, both as granting blessings.

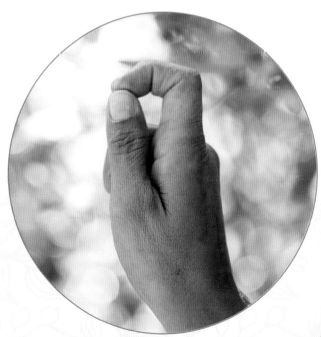

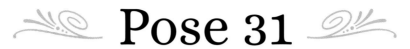

Pose 31

Mudras used for flowers

*"Where does your bounty end and where does
it begin?
You made my body out of your love and
You fed me with your own body
And you decorate my life with your beauty*

*Oh Mother Earth,
where does your bounty end and where does
it begin?
Your land has witnessed many come and go
and to each body you held and consumed
a flower has blossomed in celebration.*

*Oh Mother Earth,
where does your bounty end and where does
it begin?"*

The following mudras offer ways in which we can
embellish our practice with flowers.

Tambula mudra

Stretch your index finger and place the thumb at
the outer part of the index finger while the other
three fingers are curled at the center of the palm.

This mudra symbolizes the sprouting of seeds during
the spring season.

Pushpa mudra

Bring the thumb, index, and middle fingers together
while curling the ring and little fingers at the center of the palm. Now open up the thumb, index, and
middle fingers, revealing the blossoming of a flower.

Hamsasya mudra

This mudra represents the picking of a flower, either
to smell, offer, or place it in one's hair. Connect the
index finger with the thumb and open the other
three fingers.

Padma mudra

This mudra symbolizes a full-blown lotus flower. From
hands in prayer mudra, keep the heels of the hands
and the thumbs and little fingers connected, while
opening the ring, middle, and index fingers out in the
shape of a lotus flower.

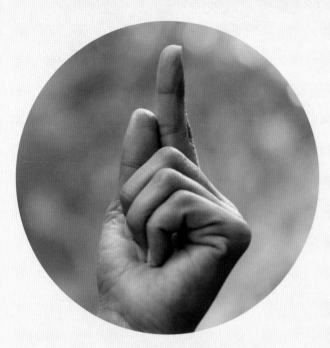

Tambula mudra

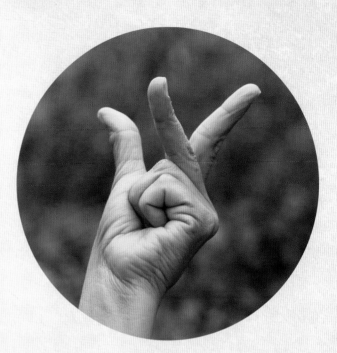

Pushpa mudra

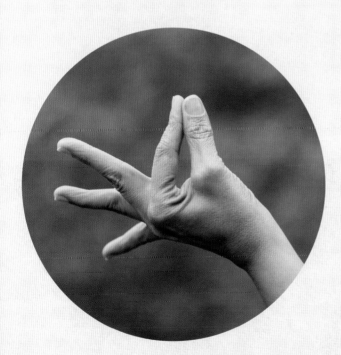

Hamsasya mudra

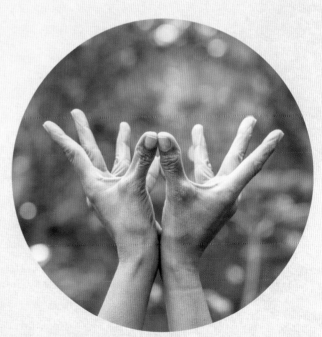

Padma mudra

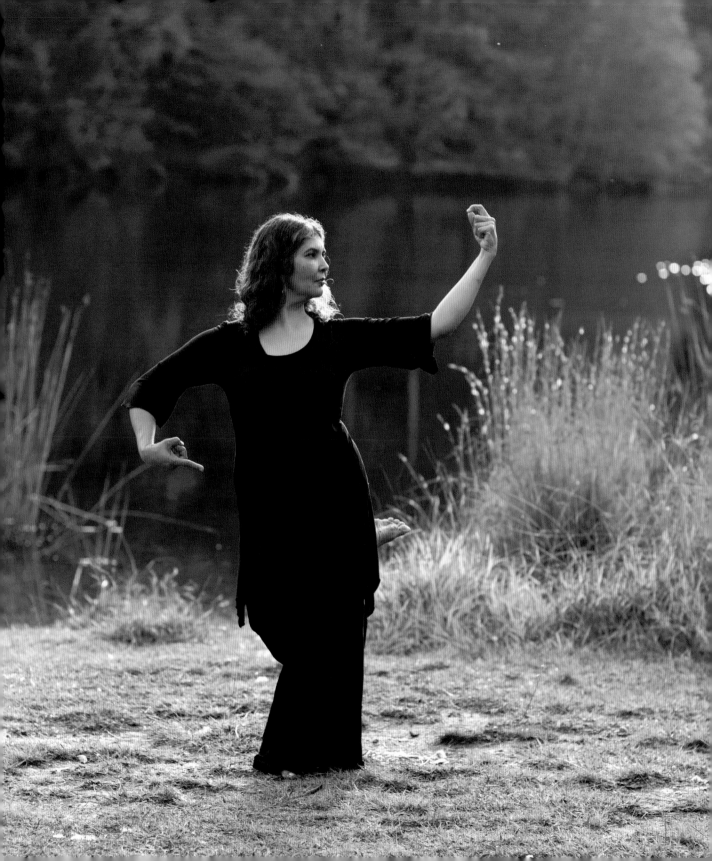

Pose 32

Standing *Sarasvati bijasana, meena puchha pada* with left hand in *kapittha mudra* and right hand in *suchi mudra*

"om aim sarasvatyai namah"

"May I flow on your riverine streams of inspiration, held by your hands of wisdom, and become capable of appreciating your art."

Mudras

For *kapittha mudra*, the thumb is traced by the index finger. This pose represents Sarasvati Devi holding the top of her celestial instrument known as the veena. For *suchi mudra*, point your index finger. The right lower hand in this pose represents Sarasvati Devi plucking the strings on her veena.

For *kapittha*, the thumb is traced by the index finger. For *suchi*, you are pointing your index finger.

Asana

This is a beautiful and feminine pose. Stand tall and turn your feet slightly out. While bending the knees, transfer the weight to the left foot, and cross the right knee behind the left knee. Look over to the left side, and point your right foot up to the sky while sitting a little deeper in the hips. Hide the right knee behind the left knee as you move the hips a few inches to the left. Now add the position of the arms and hands: The left hand is aligned with your face, and the tip of the index finger is pointing toward you. The right hand is pointing toward the center of the body, and it is held lower by the hips.

The mood for this pose is sweetness. This riverine goddess brings her waters of inspiration to cool the heat of the pain of separation. Through her music, she soothes our souls and lullabies us into remembrance and reunion.

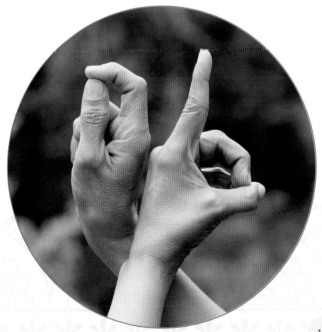

Pose 33

Seated *Sarasvati bijasana, ardha matsyendrasana* variation with left hand in *simhamukha mudra* and right hand in *sukachanchu mudra*

Mudras

In this pose, the goddess is holding her veena with a slightly different set of mudras. Her left hand at the top of her veena is in *simhamukha*, the lion's face hand gesture, with thumb and little finger pointing up while index, middle, and ring fingers are pointing straight forward toward her face. Her right hand at the bottom of her veena is in *sukachanchu*, with thumb and middle finger touching and all the other fingers circled like a wheel.

Asana

Start this pose by standing and holding your mudras. Cross your right foot in front of your left foot, leaving a foot's distance in front of the left foot and toward the left side of the body. Now come into a sitting position, bending the knees slowly and sitting on the left heel while bringing the left knee down to the floor and crossing the right leg on top of the left. If this pose is not doable, sit in *gomukhasana*, with both feet and both hips on the floor, crossing right knee over left knee.

Remember to change sides, and if you wish, you can simply place your hands in the lotus hand gesture, or *padma mudra*, on the other side.

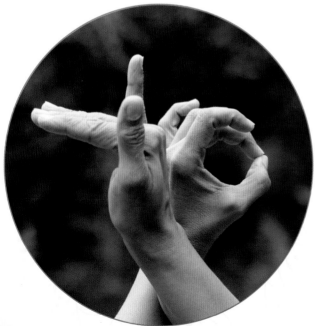

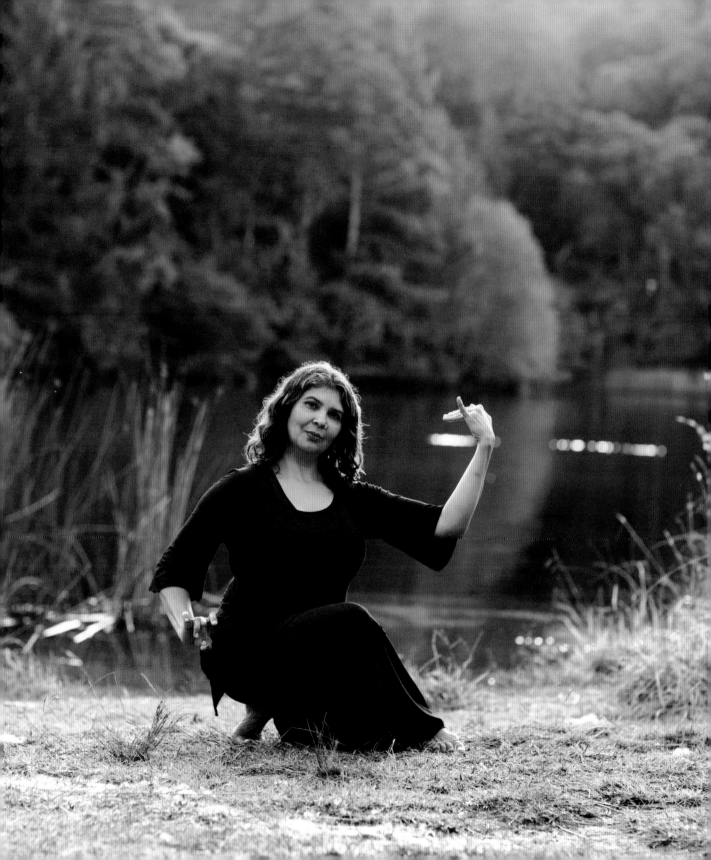

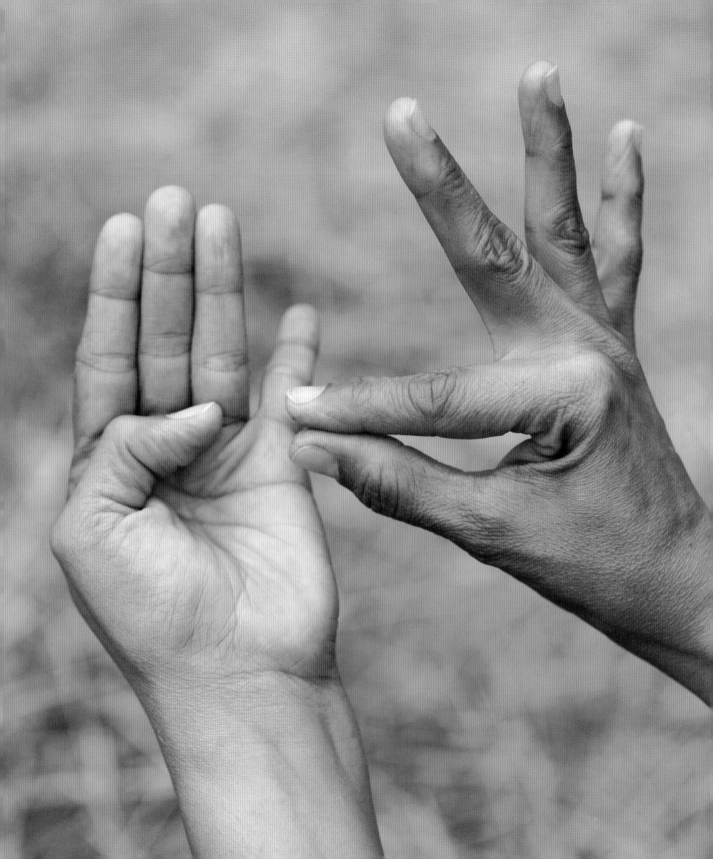

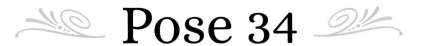

Pose 34

Brahma mudras with left hand in *chatura mudra* and right hand in *hamsasya mudra*

The left hand in *chatura mudra* becomes your sacred book. Bring the tip of the thumb to the base of the ring finger while stretching the index, middle, and ring fingers up and the little finger down. Have your palm up to the sky as the writing pad. The right hand in *hamsasya* becomes your feathery pen, as you connect the index finger and thumb and stretch the other fingers out and open.

Brahma is the energy of creation. He is the progenitor who provides us ancient knowledge. He is the beginning and the source of inspiration, creativity, and renewal. Brahma is not worshipped in Bhakti as much as the other two gods of the trinity, and yet, he is respected by all as the originating force of the universe.

Sit in meditation while holding these mudras, and from a place of emptiness, create in your mind's eye what you want to manifest. From knowledge and knowing to being and manifesting.

Pose 35

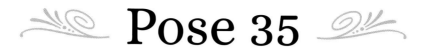

Buddha mudra or *jnana mudra*

The wisdom mudra is chosen here to represent the knowledge of the realized one, the Buddha. Buddhi is a kind of wisdom that is discerning and comes from the heart, not from the intellect. A Buddha is a person who has realized this special wisdom.

The Buddha taught us a path of nonviolence and detachment. The Buddha's teachings are called Buddha dharma, and the principles of his teachings are that we all experience suffering as humans and that we can transcend our limited human condition by awakening to our full potential as transcendental beings in these human bodies. We learn from our own experiences and grow with each other.

"sang-guie tcho-dhang tsog-kyi tchog-nam-la djang-tchub bhar-dhu dag-ni kiab-su-tchi dag-gui djin-sok guiy-pe so-nam-kyi drola phen-tchir sang-guie dru-par-shog"

"I take refuge in Buddha, dharma, and sangha until I reach enlightenment. With the practice of generosity and other perfections, may I attain Buddha's inner states for the benefit of all sentient beings."

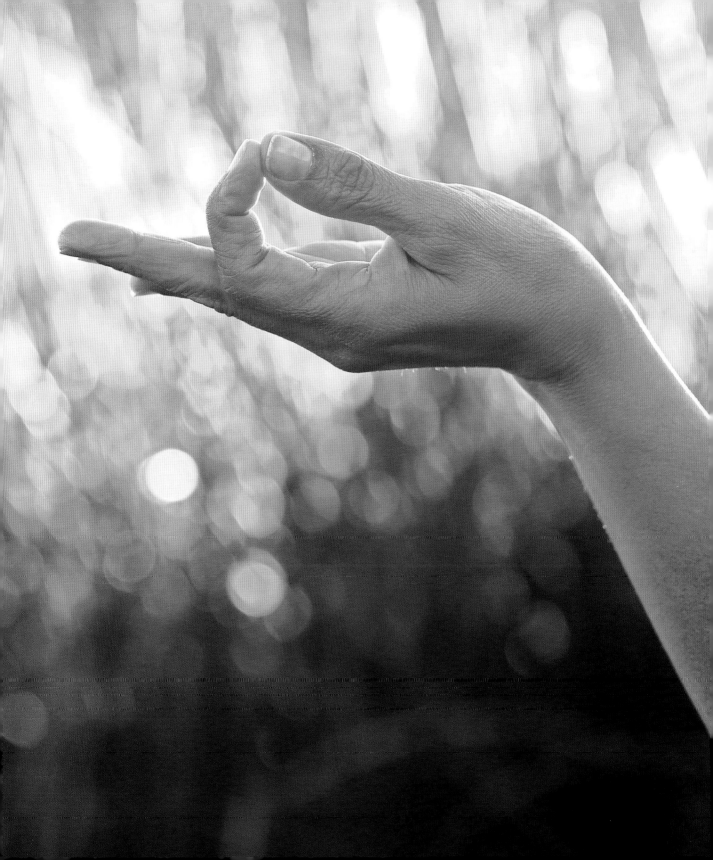

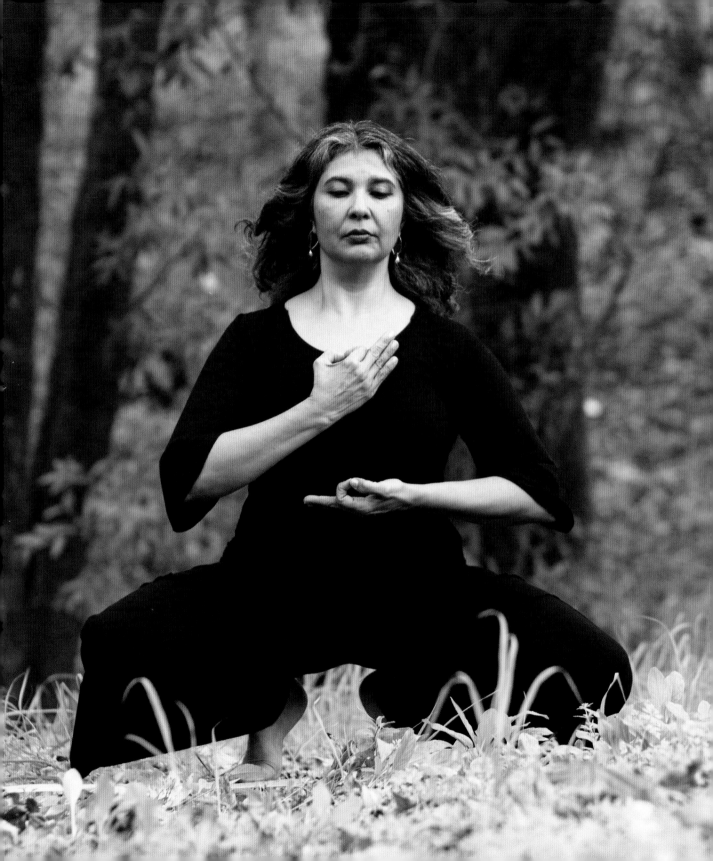

Pose 35 A

Seated *Buddha bijasana, kumbha pada* with hands in *jnana mudra*

Mudra

Bring your left hand in *jnana mudra*, connecting index finger and thumb, with your palm facing up in front of the chest. Bring your right hand in *jnana* with palm facing the heart at the center of the chest.

Asana

Come into seated *kumbha pada* on the toes or heels with your knees open. Meditate on the Buddha preaching the dharma and generously giving us a spiritual path to follow.

Pose 35 B

Walking *Buddha bijasana, rekha pada* with hands in *jnana mudra*

Mudra

Bring your left hand in *jnana mudra* with your palm facing up in front of the chest. Bring your right hand in *jnana* with palm facing the left side of the chest, above the center of your left hand, with fingers pointing up.

Asana

Walk your talk, one step at a time, aware of creating positive actions with each step.

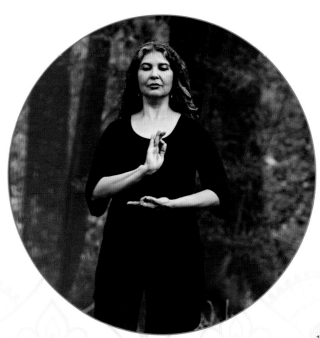

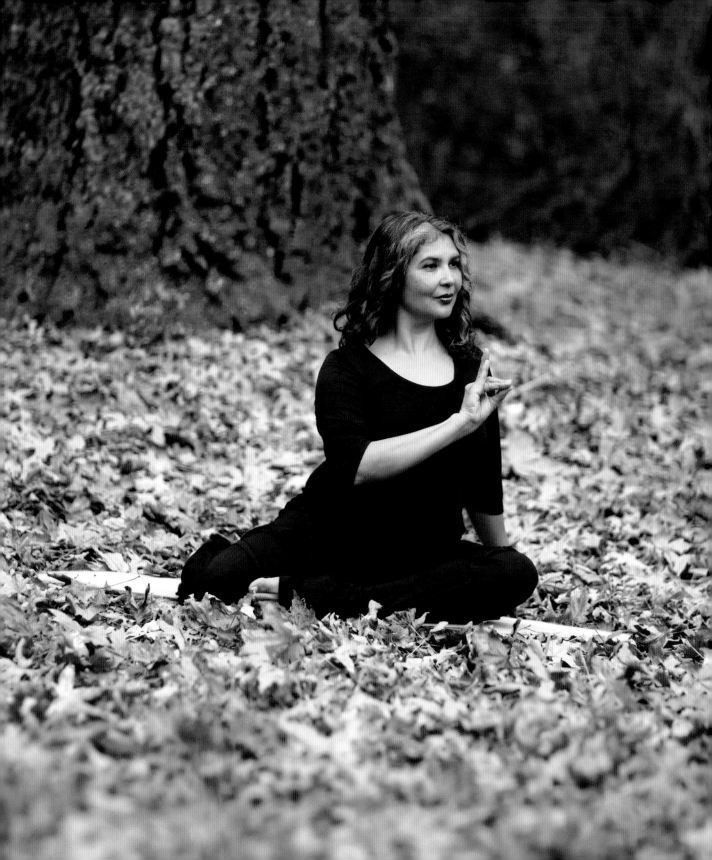

Pose 36

Mrgasana, or deer pose, with *mrgasirsa mudra*

Mudra

The deer head mudra is a very endearing hand gesture. Unite the thumb with the middle and ring fingers, and as you stretch those fingers forward, point the index and little fingers upward.

The mood of this mudra is joyful. It is one of the methods used to call the beloved.

Asana

Sit on the floor and cross the left leg in front of the body. Shift the weight to the left hip while moving the right leg back, and place the top of the right foot on the floor by the right gluteus. The right heel should be positioned by the right hip, and you can adjust the left foot to touch the right knee. Now, twist to the left by placing the left hand on the floor, as far back toward the sacrum as you can.

In your right hand, engage the deer hand gesture as you elevate your heart and your chin slightly. Internally feel the deer jumping up and down with lightness and joy, and complete the twist by placing your right hand at the heart level.

The deer is associated with Buddha in a story in which the Buddha proclaims Ahimsan—that no animals will be harmed in religious sacrifice or any circumstance.

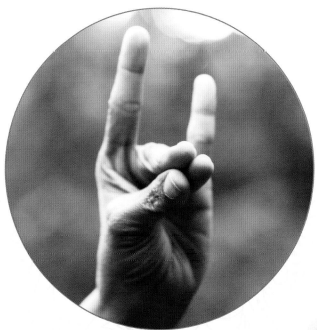

Pose 37

Kurmasana variation, or turtle pose, with Kurma mudra

About the behavior of a yogi: "One who is able to withdraw his senses from sense objects, as the tortoise draws his limbs within the shell, is to be understood as truly situated in knowledge."

—*Gita 2.58*

Mudra

This symbolic mudra, *Kurma*, shows a tortoise's shell with its four legs. The head is hidden, but you can allow it to stick out if you wish by stretching the top middle finger. Kurma, the sustainer of the universe, is one of the avatars of Vishnu.

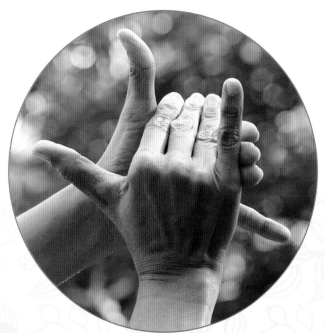

Place your hands in *simhamukha*, with the little finger and thumb pointing straight up and the other fingers moving straight forward. Then place one hand on top of the other to create a thick shell-like shape.

Asana

For this forward bend, sit on the floor, unite the soles of your feet, and move your feet far away from your hips, about 2 feet. With *Kurma mudra* in your hands, fold forward, aiming to bring your head to your feet by rounding your spine. Lift your navel up to the back body, and cave your belly. Relax your elbows on the floor, and lift your mudra. If needed, prop yourself with a bolster between your feet and head, and rest over the bolster. Forward bends provide introspection and cooling. Feel it and invite all the attention to move inward.

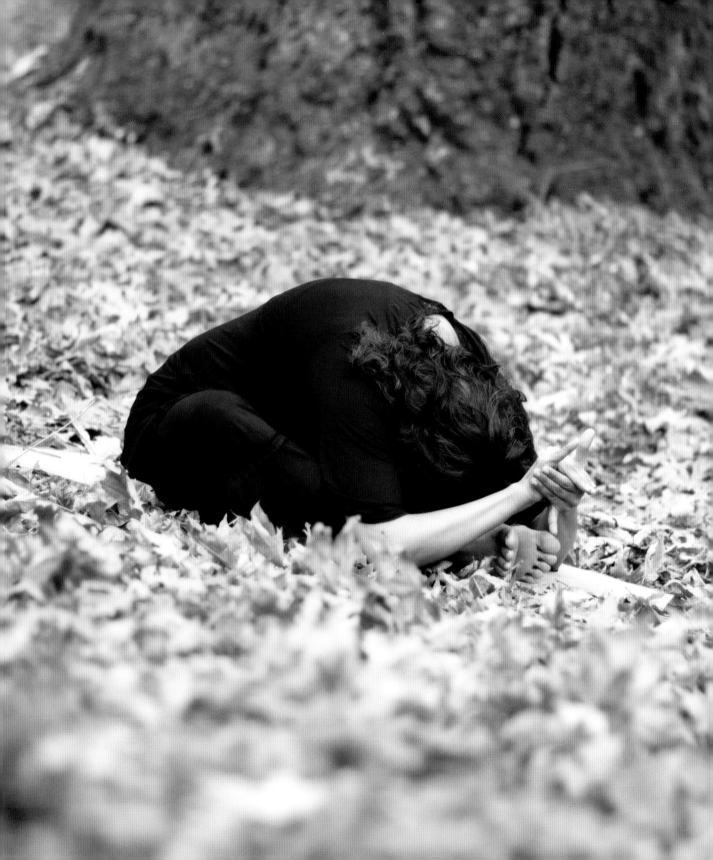

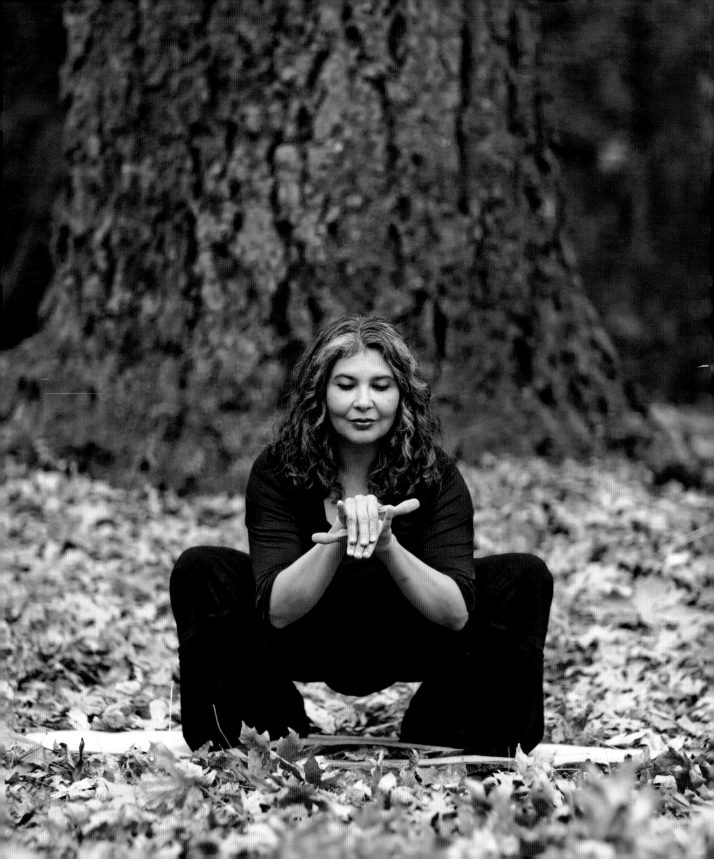

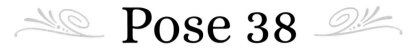

Pose 38

Malasana with *Varaha mudra*

Mudra

Another symbolic mudra for another avatar of Vishnu, Varaha takes the form of a boar. With *simhamukha mudra* once more, flatten your ring, middle, and index fingers while lifting your thumbs and little fingers. Place one hand on top of the other such that the central fingers make the snout of the boar, the little fingers form his tusks, and the thumbs form his ears. This mudra can be placed at heart level or even sometimes at face level.

Asana

Varaha saved the world by lifting it up with his tusks and rescuing everything and everyone in it. *Malasana* was chosen as a simpler pose that brings balance to the body and connects the practitioner to the earth.

The boar is constantly digging the earth with his tusks, tilling the ground, and preparing the soil for new life. Squat down with your knees, and point your feet out while slightly leaning forward and holding your *Varaha* hand gesture in front of your heart. Look inward for whatever needs to be recycled, and release it into the earth, as she will know what to do with it. Varahi, the consort of Varaha, is considered one of the most powerful mothers; she can see in the dark and purify that which cannot be seen by our ordinary eyes. If you feel strong in your legs, you can start squatting and elevate your hips a little higher than the knees to come to the full boar pose.

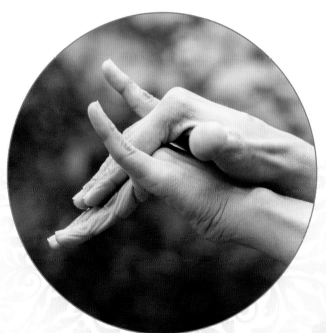

Pose 39

Salamba bhujangasana, or supported cobra,
with *nagabandha mudra*

Mudra

Two snakes coiled together form this powerful mudra. From a flat-palm *pataka mudra*, coil the tips of your fingers like snakes. Making a cross by the forearms, you will have this support, or shield, in front of your chest. This mudra can be used in a meditation pose as well to contemplate the medicine of the snakes and their association to the hidden powers of the earth.

Asana

Lie on your belly and separate your feet hip width apart while first bringing your forearms to the ground. Place your elbows below your shoulders with your palms facing down. Press the little toes and the tailbone down, connecting to the earth, while lifting the chest and the crown of the head up, like a snake lifting from the earth. After positioning the upper body upright, lift your palms in the snake hand gesture, and cross your forearms in front of your chest while balancing on your elbows, preferable on a soft, earthlike surface.

Bring to your attention your spine, and invite the energy of the Kundalini Shakti at the base of your spine to move up toward the heart center, awakening the heart and enhancing healing within the heart.

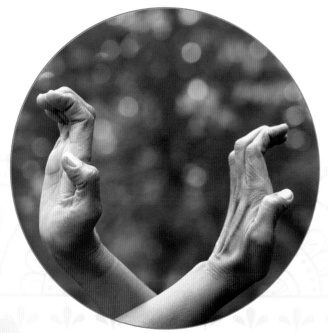

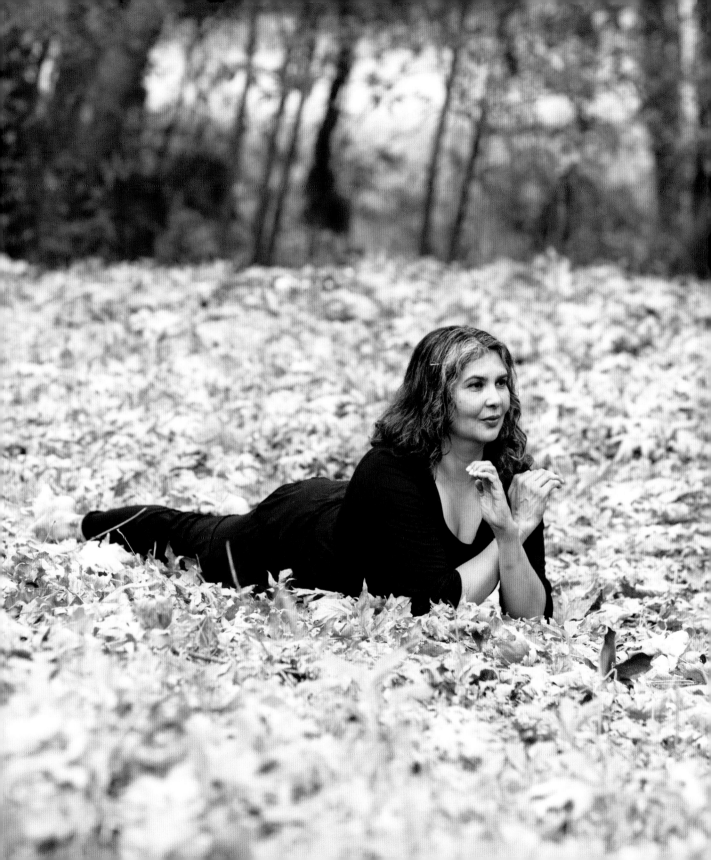

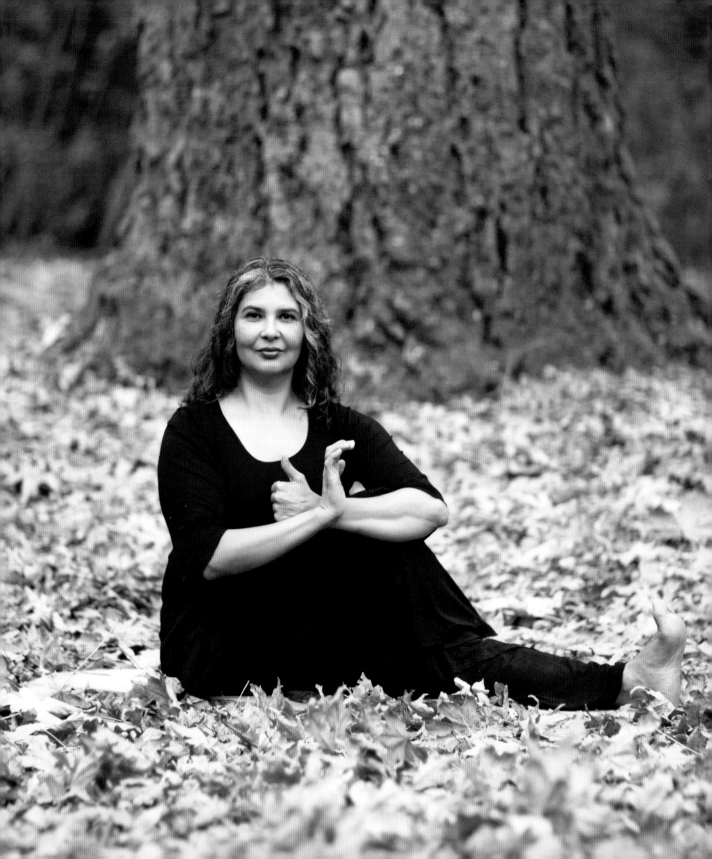

Pose 40

Matsyendrasana with sikhara and sarpasirsa mudras

Mudras

In *sikhara*, simply make a fist and move your thumb up. This hand gesture has many different meanings, like a pillar, a bow, an embrace, or the ringing of a bell. Here, this mudra represents Shiva in his archetypal symbol as the lingam, or phallus.

For *sarpasirsa*, bring your flat palm to a snakelike shape by bending the fingers in a curved line at the top. In this storytelling this hand gesture is showing another symbol or power of Shiva: the snake coiled around the Shiva lingam.

Asana

Seated on the ground, stretch your legs forward in *dandasana* while keeping your spine straight. Bend your right knee, and cross your right foot over to the left side of your thigh. Press the sole of the right foot on the ground while bringing your left arm around your right leg and twisting your upper body to the right. Bring your left hand to *sikhara*, and bring your right hand to the ground by the sacrum, while looking over to the right shoulder. Keep the torso twisted, and shift your gaze to the center of your heart. Now bring your right hand to *sarpasirsa*, crossing at the wrists.

Matsyendranath was a follower of Shiva, and all of the hatha yogis of the past were part of the Nath cult. These two mudras, together with the trisula, or trident, honor Shiva's lineage.

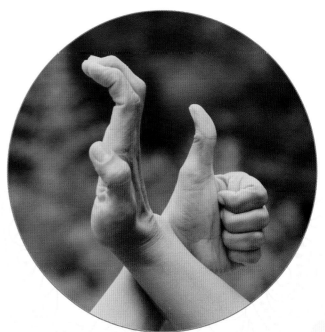

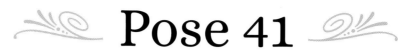

Pose 41

Vasishthasana with *sarpasirsa mudra*

Mudra

The *sarpasirsa mudra*, or the serpent hand gesture, is used in this abhinaya again to honor Lord Shiva, the one who wears snakes as his garlands. Sage Vasishtha was a very honorable master, and like many other sages, he worshipped Shiva. Vasishtha's main teachings were compiled and written by Sage Vyasa in a text titled *Yoga Vasishtha* that described the conversation between Vasishtha and his disciple, Lord Rama.

Asana

Vasishthasana is a pose that requires focus and strength. Come onto hands and knees, and align the left shoulder over the left hand as you begin to open your torso to the right, lifting your right arm up toward the sky and stretching the right leg to place the arch of your right foot in alignment with the left knee. You can stay in this variation of *ardha vasishthasana*, or you can stretch the left leg as well by placing the left foot in front of the right foot and turning the chest up toward the sky. Now add the serpent mudra to your right hand.

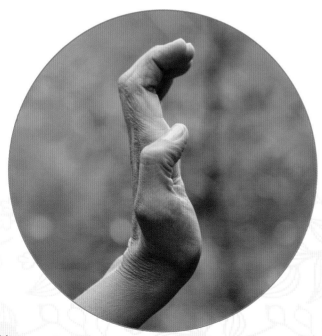

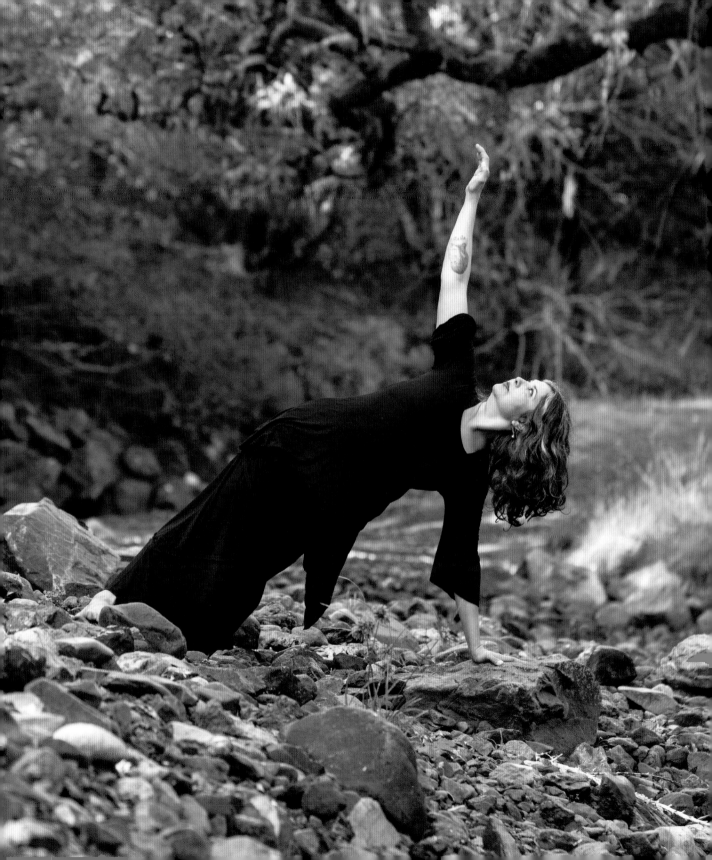

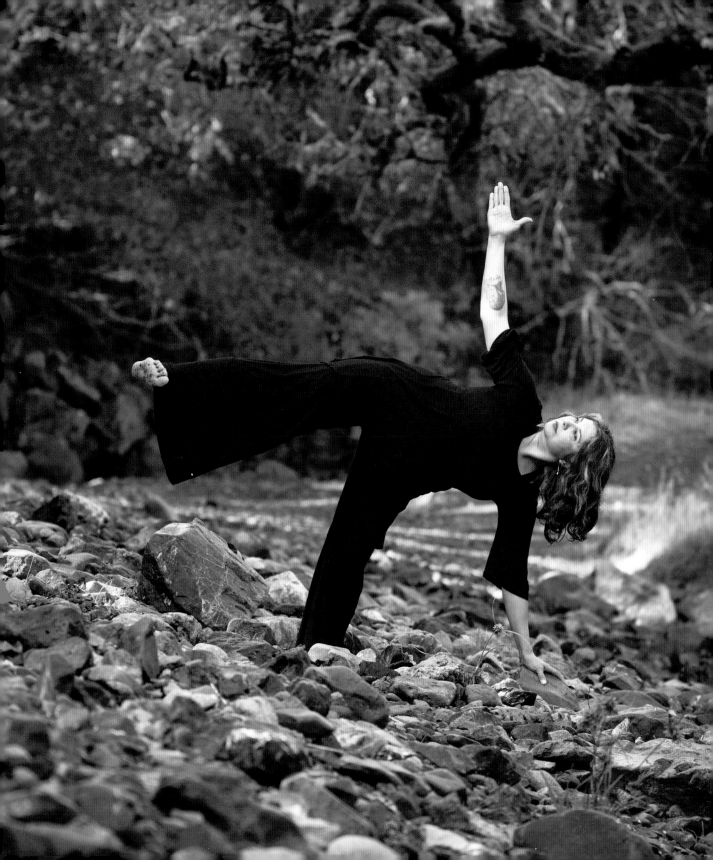

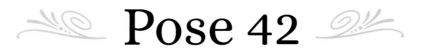

Pose 42

Ardhachandrasana with *ardhachandra mudra*

Mudra

Ardhachandra, or half-moon hand gesture, is used in this pose to match the half-moon asana. In this mudra, the palm is flat, and the thumb is open to the side, making the shape of the half-moon between the index finger and the thumb.

Another mudra that can be used with this pose is *chandrakala*, the digit of the moon. Open your palm in *ardhachandra*, and then fold in the little, ring, and middle fingers, pointing only the index finger upward and the thumb sideways.

Asana

Start with a standing pose, and fold halfway down. Stay halfway down, and place your left finger pads underneath the left shoulders; some of you can place the left hand on a block or, if you can do this in nature like I did, use a higher rock. Begin to open your right arm up to the sky while lifting your right leg up to hip height and turning the toes out to the right. Shift the gaze to right hand, and place your hands in *ardhachandra* hand gesture.

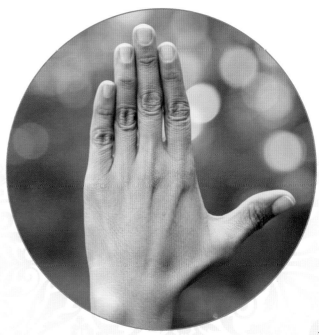

Pose 43

Virabhadrasana three with *trisula mudra*

Mudra

Trisula is the trident and one of Shiva's weapons. Simply connect the thumb to the little finger, and spread the three central fingers, showing the three points of the trident. Shiva's trisula is said to operate in the three worlds, or *triloka*: the physical plane or Bhuloka, the subtle plane or Antarloka, and the causal plane or Sivaloka. Shiva's gift of destruction of ego will be effective in all planes of existence.

Asana

Stand tall in mountain pose, and engage your hands in *trisula mudra*. Lift your left hand or arm up to the sky while keeping your right hand with the *trisula* pointing down. Begin to lean forward while lifting your right leg up, eventually bringing your torso and right leg parallel to the ground. Keep the head aligned with the left arm, and gaze at a chosen spot on the ground.

Virabhadra is a powerful warrior who was born out of one of Shiva's dreadlocks in a moment of Shiva's fury against King Daksha for unintentionally provoking Sati, Shiva's first Shakti, who threw herself into the fire to die. Daksha was Sati's father, and he was very unhappy with his daughter marrying the yogi Shiva. To make his point, and with the intention to ostracize Shiva, Daksha created a huge ritual celebration, *yagna*, and did not invite the *maha* yogi. When Sati discovered this, she offered herself into sacrificial fire, leaving this world to be reborn as Parvati.

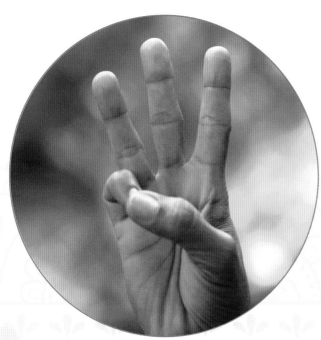

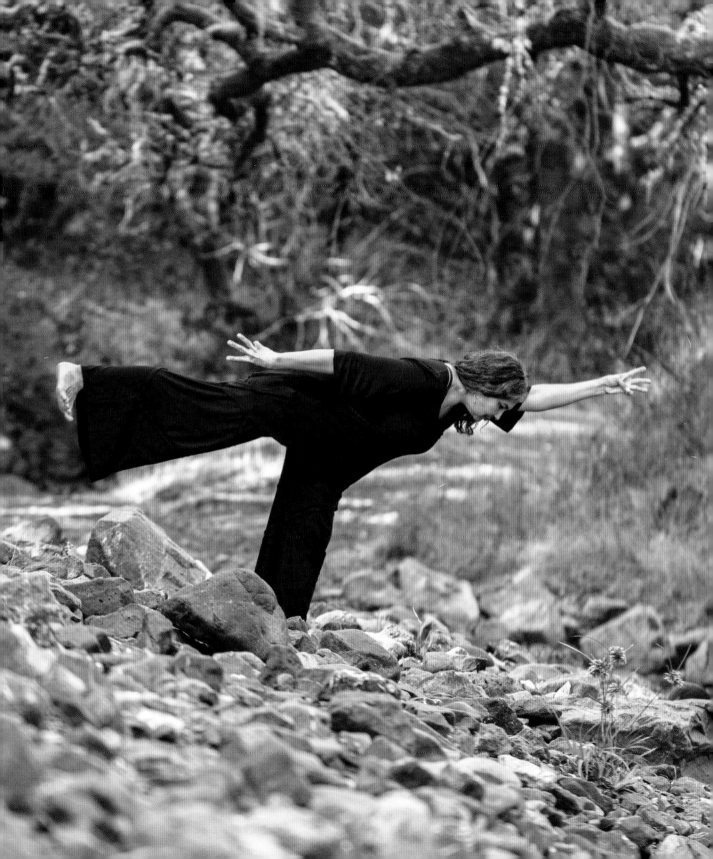

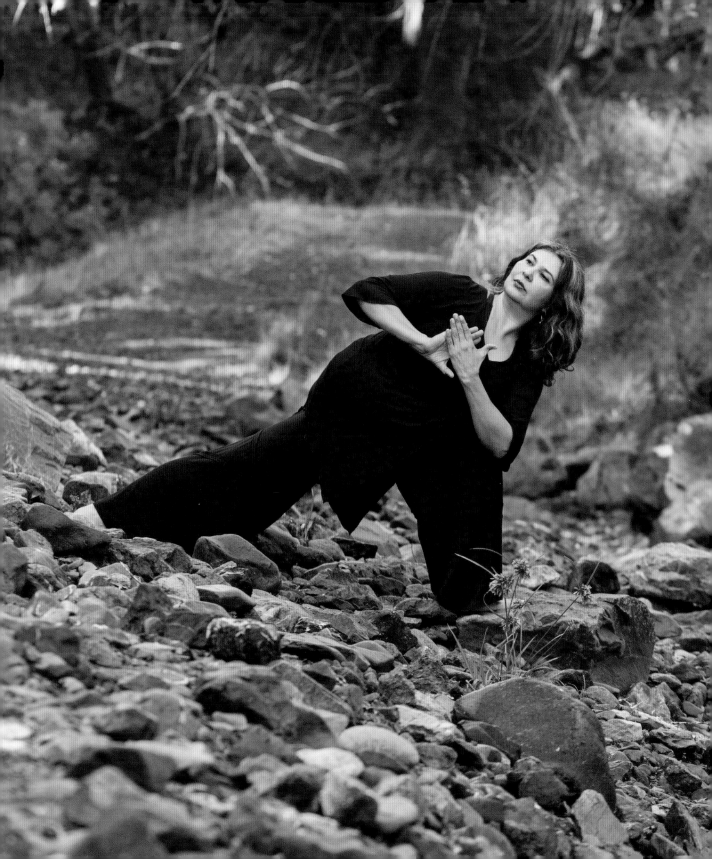

Pose 44

Parivritta parsvakonasana with *chakra mudra*

Mudra

Open your hands in *ardhachandra mudra*, and place the centers of the palms together, with the tips of the fingers and thumbs pointing to the four directions resembling the movement of a wheel. The *chakra mudra* here represents one of Mother Durga's weapons. In order to help kill the demon Mahisasura, Sri Vishnu gifted Mother Durga his own discus, Shiva gave her his own trident, Varuna gave her his conch, and Agni presented her with his spear.

The discus chakra will destroy from afar whatever evil is coming your way before it comes too close.

Asana

Stand tall and separate your feet 3.5 feet apart. Turn your right foot out 90 degrees and your left foot in 45 degrees. Bend your right knee 90 degrees, pointing that knee toward the right middle toe. Twist your torso to bring your left elbow to the outer knee while powering the left inner thigh to move back and up by pressing the outer edge of the left foot down. Point your right arm up toward the sky, and look toward your right hand in order to lift the torso and twist deeper. Now bring your head to a neutral position, and place your hands in the *chakra mudra* right in front of the heart.

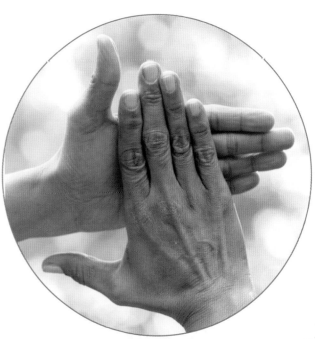

Pose 45

Skandasana one with *mayura mudra*

Mudra

Bring your right hand to *kapittha mudra* by bringing the index finger to touch the right thumb—this is the body of the peacock. Now open your left palm, stretching the fingers away from each other to create the circle of the open feathers of the peacock. To complete the mudra, place the back of your right hand at the center of your left palm.

Asana

Stand with your feet 3 to 4 feet apart, depending on how tall you are. Turn your feet out, and begin to bend the right knee, coming to a squat-like shape on the right leg while lifting the left toes and balancing on the left heel. It is OK if the right heel does not touch the ground; it will just require a little more balance. For an easier variation, you can stop with your right knee bent at a 90-degree angle. The final part is to add the mudra, which represents Skanda's vehicle, the peacock.

There is an endearing story in which Skanda and Ganesha, as brothers tend to do, were fighting to see who would win their parents' attention. Some sweets were also part of the dispute. They decided that whoever was able to go around the world three times the fastest would win. Skanda jumped on his peacock and flew away, while Ganesha slowly circumambulated Shiva and Parvati, winning the game by declaring that the divine couple represented the entire universe. Skanda's agility was defeated by Ganesha's intelligence.

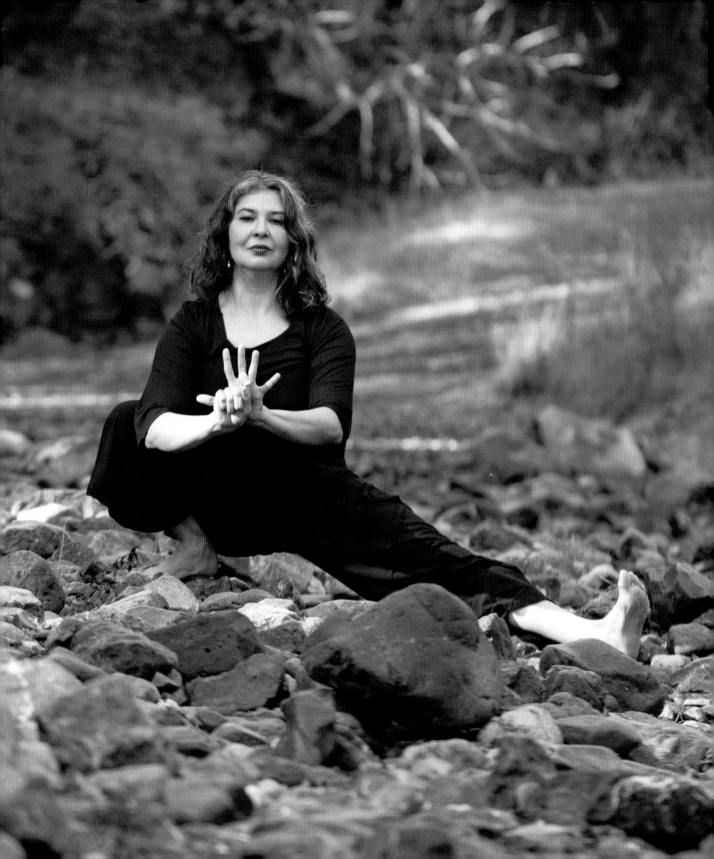

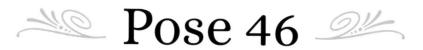

Pose 46

Skandasana two with two hands in *musti mudra*

Mudra

Musti for *skandasana* symbolizes strength and in this story shows how Skanda is holding his main weapon, the spear. While bringing your hands into a fist, imagine that you are holding this fast and sharp spear.

Asana

Stand tall and separate your feet about 3 feet apart. Turn your feet out and bend the left knee, coming to a squat on the left side while lifting the right toes up. Bend the side slightly to the left while adding the hand gesture of holding the spear and looking over to the right side.

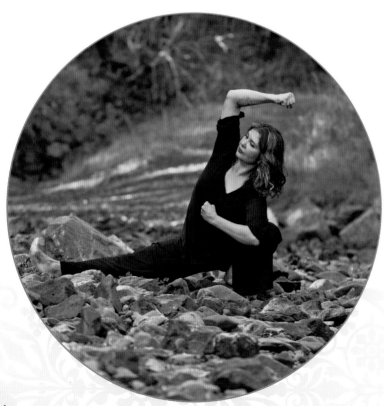

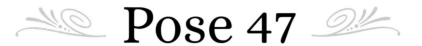

Pose 47

Parivritta navasana with two hands in *musti mudra*

Mudra

Musti for *parivritta navasana*, revolving boat pose, symbolizes the focus and the strength of rolling a boat. When holding this mudra, imagine holding the oar and rowing a boat.

Asana

Sit on the floor and bend your knees, bringing the hands to the outer knees, and lean back while balancing on your hips and lifting your chest and feet to knee height. Once you feel balanced and solid, add a twist to the right, and add the *musti mudras*. When twisting to the right, lift your left arm higher than the right, and when twisting to the left, lift your right arm higher than the left.

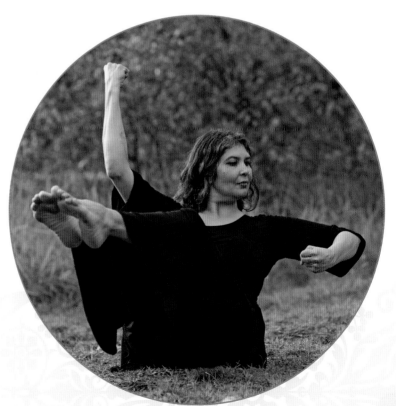

Pose 48

Utthita trikonasa with *katakamukha mudra*

Mudra

Katakamukha one is a mudra used a lot in the pure dance style. It has different variations and many different meanings. The literal translation is "the opening of a bracelet," and it can be used to pick up flowers, to prepare sandal paste, or to reveal the feelings in one's heart. This *hasta* is used to draw the string of a bow like in the next pose, *virabhadrasana two*. Here in this pose, we are using this *katakamukha* simply to decorate this asana.

Bring to touch your thumb, index, and middle fingers, and stretch them forward, making a sharp, beak-like shape while stretching the ring and pinkie fingers slightly up like the rays of the sun.

Asana

Stand tall with your feet 3 to 3.5 feet apart. Turn your right foot out 90 degrees, and turn your left heel out to a 45-degree angle. Firm the legs by lifting the kneecaps and engaging the muscles of the thighs. Align the right side of the body with the right leg, and open the right thigh out while spiraling the left thigh inward. Bring your hands to *katakamukha one* as you lift your arms up to shoulder height and lean over to the right side to bring your torso parallel to the ground. As you do this, keep the hips still, and open your torso to the sky.

This mudra was chosen here in honor of the Bharatanatyam style of dance.

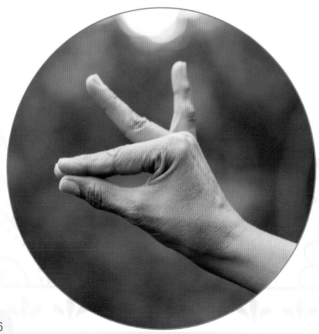

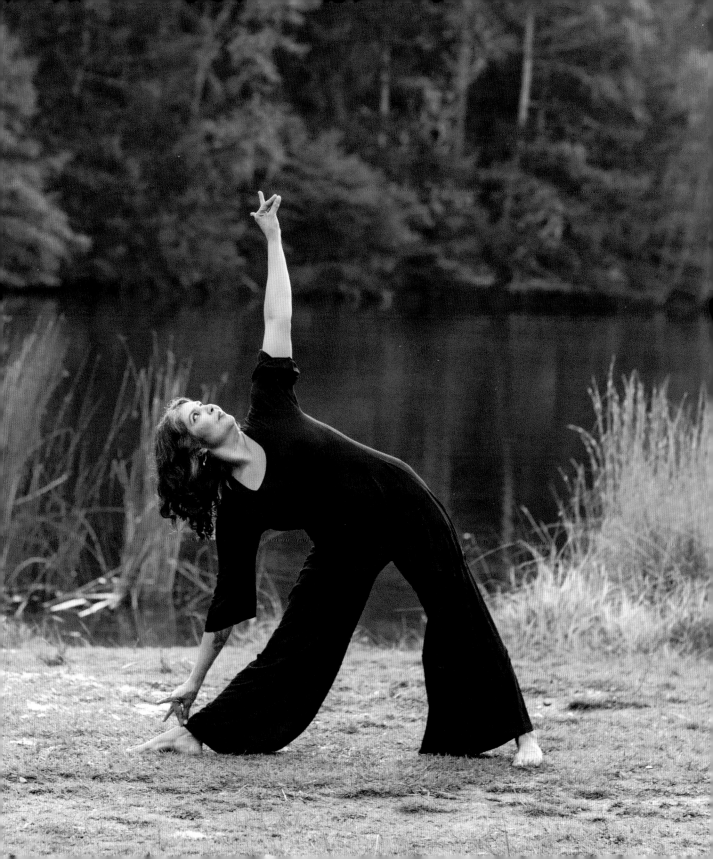

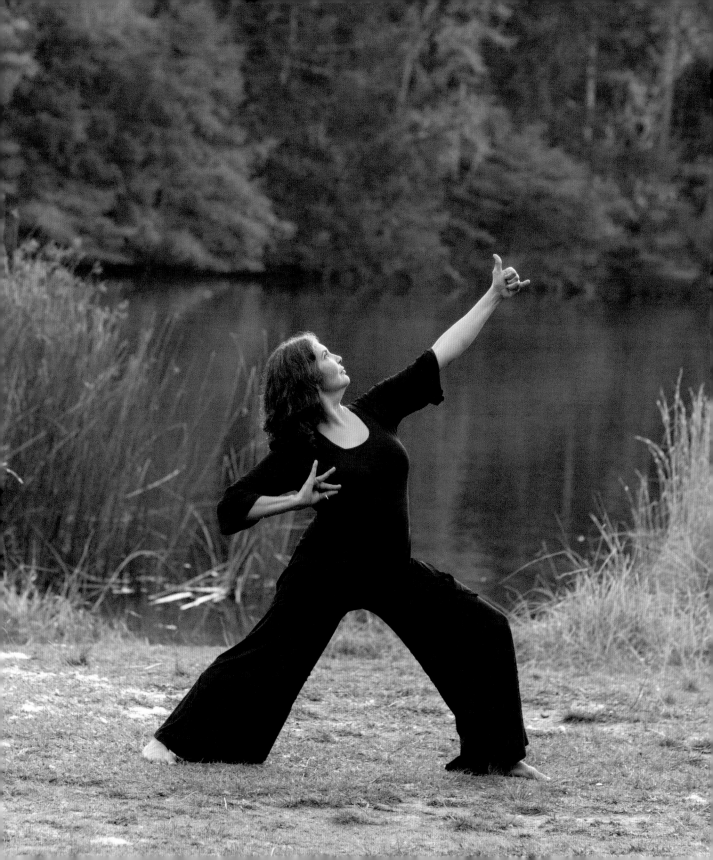

Pose 49

Virabhadrasana two with *dhanu* and *katakamukha one mudras*

Mudras

Katakamukha can be initiated by bringing all the fingers in one hand together in *mukula mudra* and slowly opening the little finger and the ring finger away from the other three.

For *dhanu* hand gesture, bring the index, middle, and ring fingers to touch the heel of your palm while stretching the thumb and pinkie away from the center of the palm and away from each other. During this hand gesture, make sure to bend the wrists a little bit in such a way that the palms move toward your forearms slightly.

Asana

Standing with your feet about 3.5 feet apart, turn your right foot 90 degrees out to the right and your left foot 45 degrees inward. Bend your left knee over your left heel while pointing the left knee toward the middle toe. Keep the outer edge of the right foot pressing down to the ground, and power the right inner leg to move backward and upward.

First, open your arms to the sides with your hands in *pataka* at shoulder height. Then, while looking over your left hand, engage *dhanu mudra*. While bringing your right hand to heart level, place it in *katakamukha one*, and imagine that you are stringing the bow as you either continue looking forward, or look slightly upward to the sky.

We are giving this warrioress a bow and an arrow, but you could give her a sword like Kali's, or you could have your left hand in *musti* as if you are holding a shield while slightly bending that elbow to hold the shield closer to you heart.

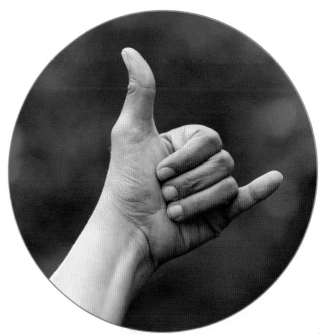

Pose 50

Utthita janurhastasana with *suchi mudra*

Mudra

Suchi is a beautiful hand gesture that shows us the oneness in everything and everyone. This asana is showing us the one-pointed focus of support that, in the practice of yoga, is called *ekagrata*. *Suchi*, among many different meanings, points to the holding of the discus or chakra. Simply stretch your index finger while connecting the thumb to the other remaining fingers.

Asana

In this simple balance position, we practice unevenness to strengthen our balance. Come off center on one leg to find equilibrium within challenge. Stand tall in *tadasana*, mountain pose, and as you ground yourself through your right foot, lift your left knee to meet your left hand while bringing your left hand to hold your left kneecap. Now lift your right hand in *suchi* hand gesture at the level of your eyes, and concentrate on the index finger while grounding through the right foot and extending the crown of your head upward.

This asana can be done in a more advanced variation with left hand holding the left big toe and the left leg straight in *utthita padangusthasana*.

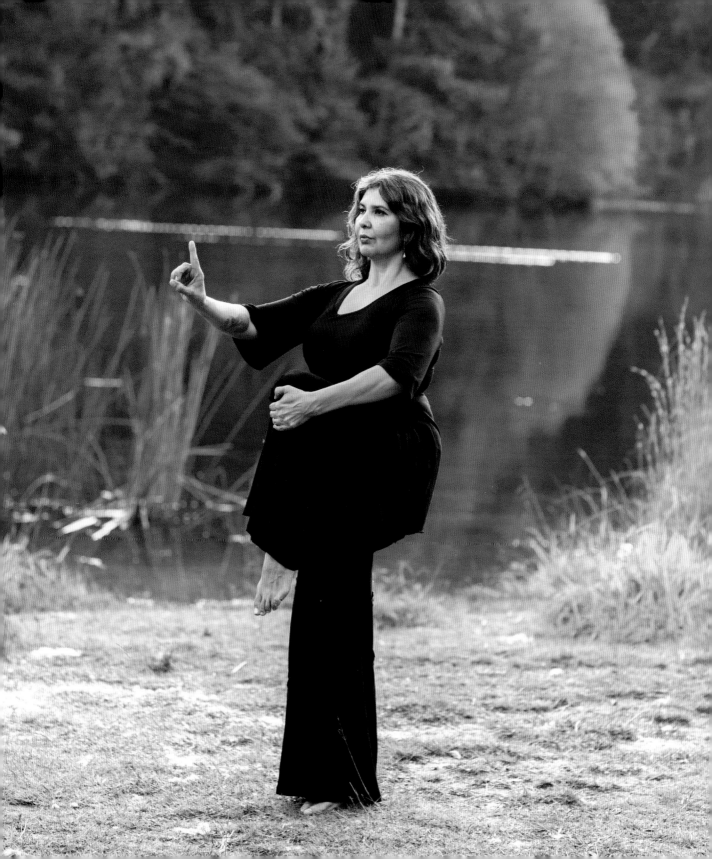

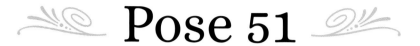

Pose 51

Navasana with *alapadma mudra*

Mudra

Alapadma hand gesture can be combined with many asanas, and in the art of hand gestures and story-telling, it has many different meanings. For the mudrasana combination, we will be focusing on it as symbolizing either the rays of the sun or a fire.

Open your palm, and hold it facing up. Now stretch the fingers like the rays of the sun. Keep the thumb by the base of the index finger, point the index finger forward, keep the middle finger higher than the index finger, position the ring finger higher than the middle finger, and hold the little finger higher than the ring finger. You can imagine a fiery ball, like a small sun, in your palm, with the fingers symbolizing the rays of that sun.

Asana

Navasana, or boat pose, is another balance pose that awakens strength not only in the lower body but also at the center of the body. Start by sitting on the ground, and bend the knees, bringing the hands to the back of the knees and leaning back a little, enough to lift your feet slightly up and find balance on your hips. Avoid balancing on your sacrum—if you went that far back, return to a more upright posi-tion. Lift your heart center up, and stretch your arms forward with your hands in *alapadma*, palms up to the sun. Either stay in this variation, or stretch the legs forward and up and lift your arms a little higher toward the sky, connecting to the sun.

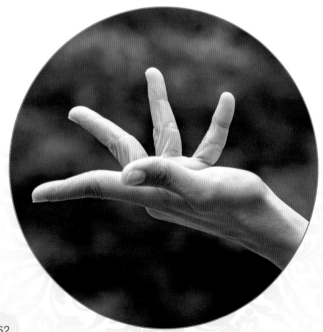

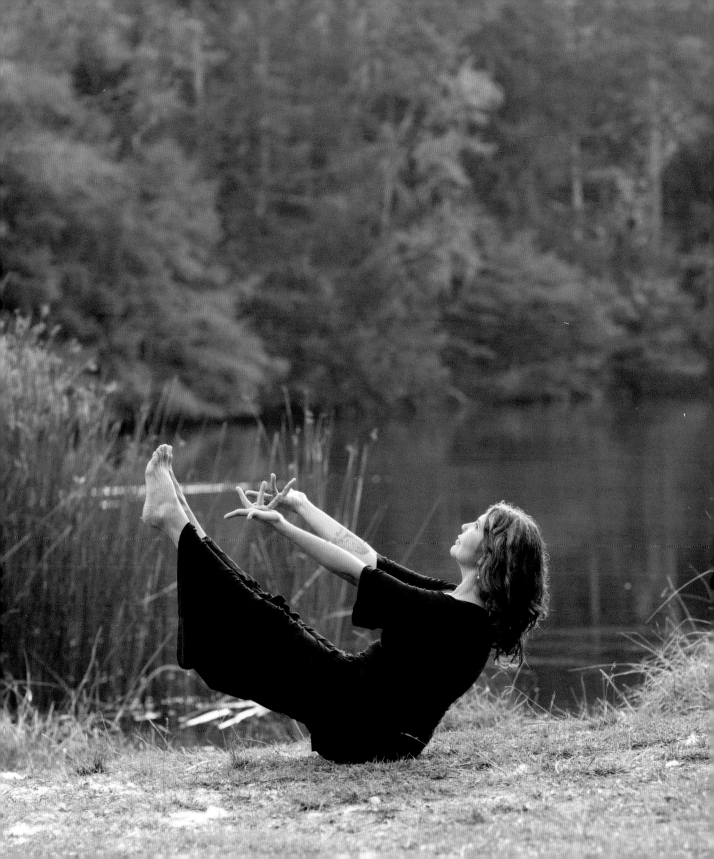

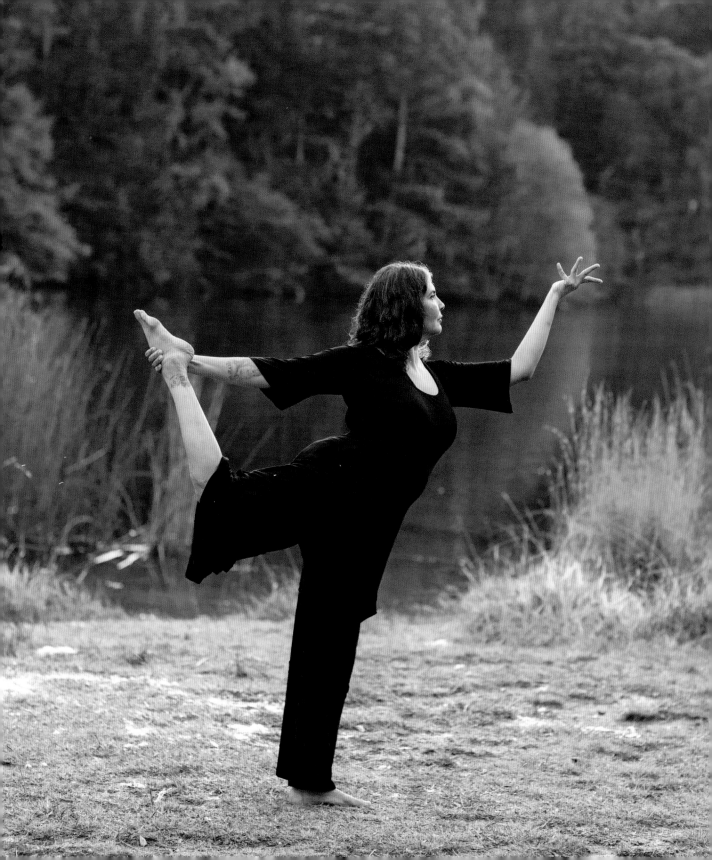

Pose 52

Natarajasana or *pinakinasana* with *alapadma mudra*

Mudra

Alapadma hand gesture can be combined with many asanas, and in the art of hand gestures and story-telling, it has many different meanings. For the mudrasana combination, we will be focusing on it as symbolizing either the rays of the sun or a fire.

Open your palm, and hold it facing up. Now stretch the fingers like the rays of the sun. Keep the thumb by the base of the index finger, point the index finger forward, keep the middle finger higher than the index finger, position the ring finger higher than the middle finger, and hold the little finger higher than the ring finger. You can imagine a fiery ball, like a small sun, in your palm, with the fingers symbolizing the rays of that sun.

Asana

Stand tall and ground yourself through the four corners of the left foot while moving your right foot back and up to hold the outer edge of the right foot with your right hand. Move your knee in to align with your hip, and lean forward, looking to your left hand as you stretch your arm forward, and add *alapadma mudra* to this pose. As you find a balance, come to a more upright position by kicking the right foot back and lifting your hand to align with your face so that you can gaze at the fire in your hands.

This balance position, associated with Lord Shiva, in traditional hatha yoga came to be called *natarajasana*, or "Shiva the dancer." If we follow the scriptures, Shiva during his tandava dance is using a different set of hand gestures and a different pose, so in my school of yoga, I call this pose *pinakinasana*, referring to Shiva, also known as Pinakin, the one who is armed with the *pinaka* bow.

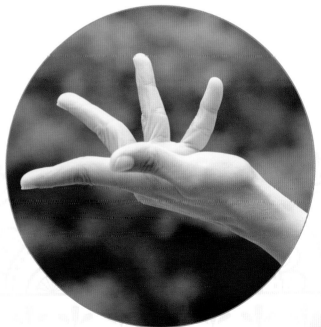

Pose 53

Utthita hasta padangusthasana with *alapadma mudra*

Mudra

Alapadma hand gesture can be combined with many asanas, and in the art of hand gestures and story-telling, it has many different meanings. For the mudrasana combination, we will be focusing on it as symbolizing either the rays of the sun or a fire.

Open your palm, and hold it facing up. Now stretch the fingers like the rays of the sun. Keep the thumb by the base of the index finger, point the index finger forward, keep the middle finger higher than the index finger, position the ring finger higher than the middle finger, and hold the little finger higher than the ring finger. You can imagine a fiery ball, like a small sun, in your palm, with the fingers symbolizing the rays of that sun.

Asana

From standing, come to balance on your left foot while lifting your right knee up to the chest. Stretch your right leg forward, either using a scarf around your right foot for support or holding your right big toe with your right hand. Keep the hips even. It does not matter how high you can lift your right leg—the most important part is to stay centered. Now stretch your left arm in front of you with your hand in *alapadma* hand gesture while lifting your chest and connecting your heart to the rays of the sun in your hands and all around you. You can keep your gaze on your hand while feeling your entire body being alive and your foot firmly rooted on the earth.

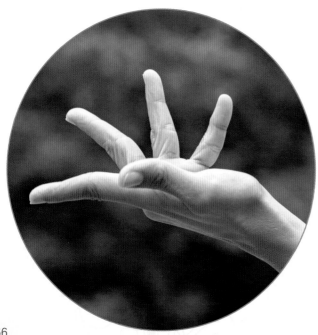

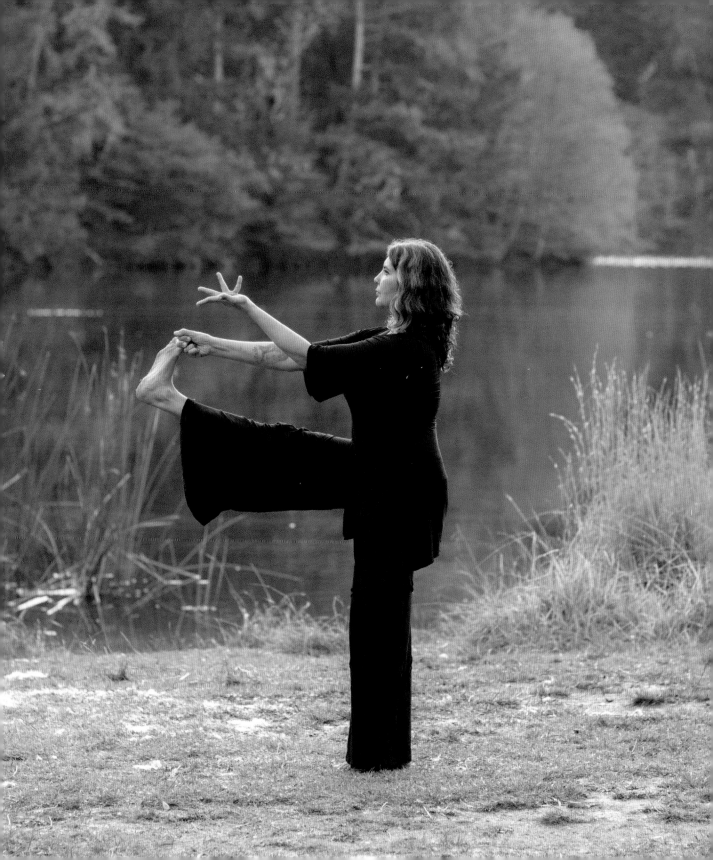

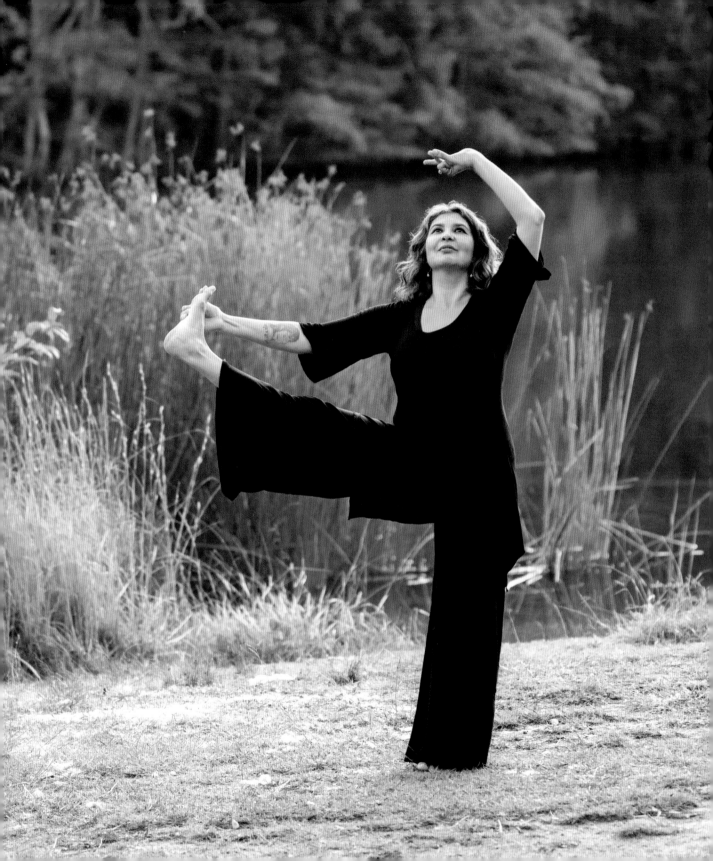

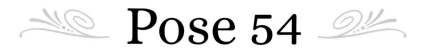

Pose 54

Utthita hastapada with bhramara mudra

Mudra

Bhramara, the bee mudra, is a symbolic and poetic hand gesture. Bring the tip of your index finger to the inner base of your thumb, and now connect the tip of the middle finger to the tip of the thumb while separating and stretching the ring and little fingers away from the other fingers.

The high vibration of a bee, its sounds, and its effects in our environment mean that the bee hand gesture is associated with the crown chakra and higher realms.

Bhramari is the goddess of the bees, and she is associated with Mother Parvati. You can use the *bhramara mudra* in meditation as well and call upon Bhramari Devi's strength and power.

Asana

Stand with even weight on both feet, and engage *bhramara mudra* in your left hand. Keep your arm relaxed and down for now. Lift your right foot up, and use a belt to support stretching the right leg out to the side. Alternatively, you may hold the outer edge of the right foot as you open your right leg out. Keep the hips even and down as you lift the leg and find your balance by gazing at a central line. Now lift your bee hand gesture above your head, and if you can, shift your gaze to your hand.

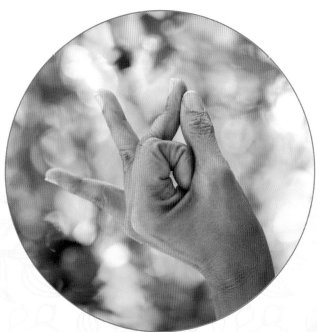

Pose 55

Parivritta utthita hastapada with *darpana mudra*

Mudra

Darpana means "mirror." The hand is a simple *pataka hasta*; the only difference is that you place the palm in front of your face like a mirror. The bend of the limbs is a big part of the beautiful choreography of Odissi dance, so when doing the mirror hand gesture, make sure to bend at the wrist and elbows.

Sometimes I ask my students to look into the *darpana mudra* as a meditation—to look at their own reflection, find their inner beauty, and work to see that same reflection of beauty and light in others.

Asana

Our last balance pose is a twist. Stand tall on both feet, and lift your left knee up. Either place a strap around your left foot and hold the strap with the right hand, or hold the outer edge of the left foot with your right hand. Look forward, and stretch the left leg forward and up. Keep the hips even and squared. Now place your left hand on your sacrum, the triangle bone at the base of your spine, and twist to the left. You can stay in this variation, or you can turn your gaze back by aligning your chin with your left shoulder, stretching the left arm back, and adding the mirror hand gesture. Look right inside the center of your palm.

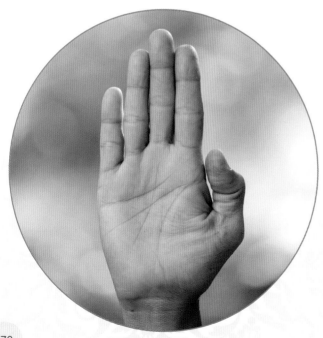

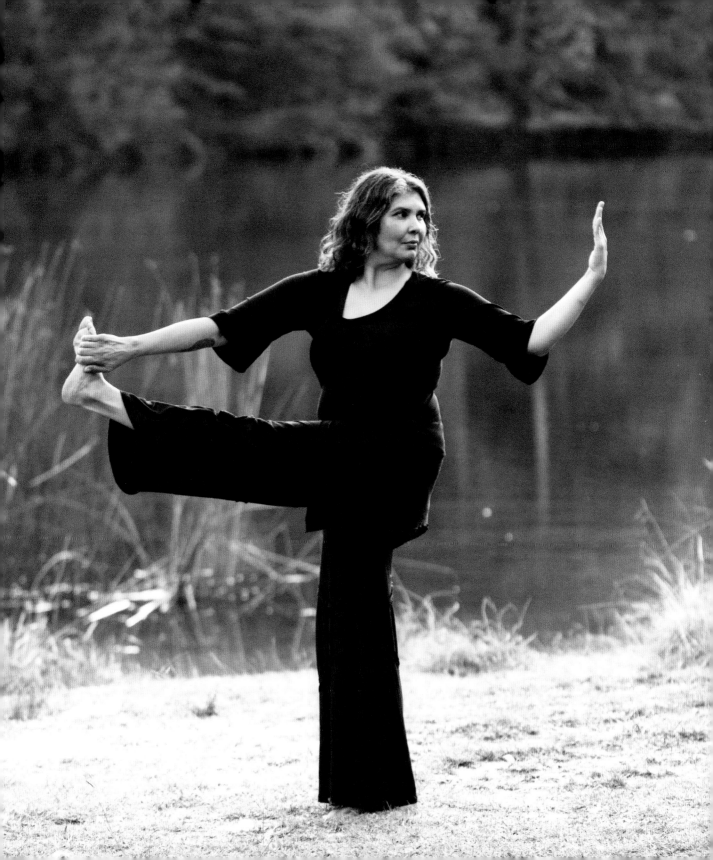

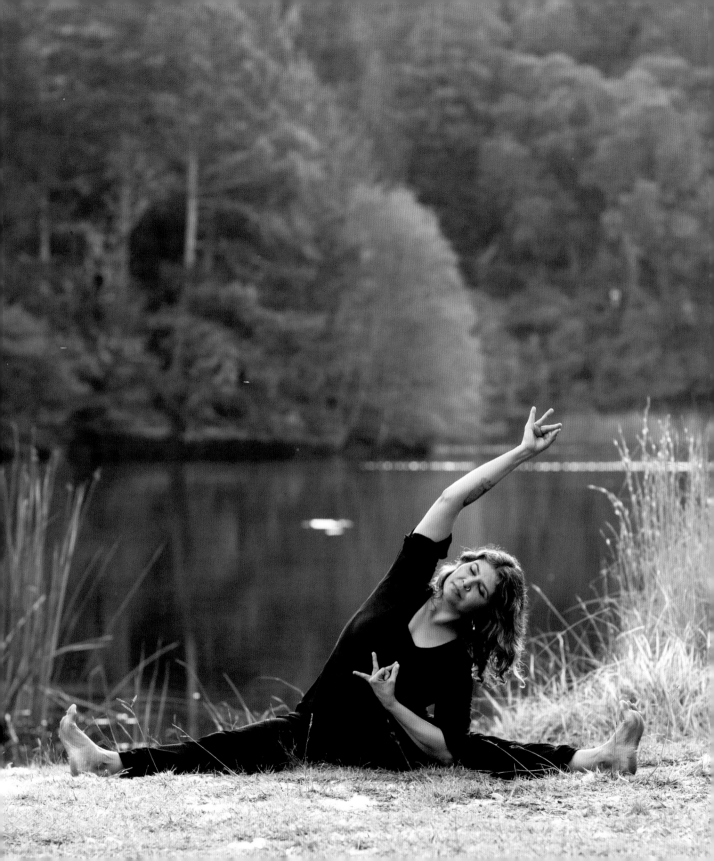

Pose 56

Parshva upavishta konasana with bhramara mudra

Mudra

Bhramara, the bee mudra, is a symbolic and poetic hand gesture. Bring the tip of your index finger to the inner base of your thumb, and now connect the tip of the middle finger to the tip of the thumb while separating and stretching the ring and little fingers away from the other fingers.

The high vibration of a bee, its sounds, and its effects in our environment mean that the bee hand gesture is associated with the crown chakra and higher realms.

Bhramari is the goddess of the bees, and she is associated with Mother Parvati. You can use the *bhramara mudra* in meditation as well and call upon Bhramari Devi's strength and power.

Asana

Connecting to the earth by sitting down, stretch your legs out to the sides at a comfortable distance where you can still keep your hips moving down and you are not compressing the bones on your hip joints. Move the muscles of your gluteus back, and make sure to sit on your sitting bones. Some of you can benefit from elevating the hips with a blanket.

Bring your hands to the bee hand gesture, *bhramara mudra*, and rest your hands on your legs for a moment while lifting the heart and the crown upward. Now lift your right arm up, and as you side-bend to the left, bring your right arm over your head with arm and ear aligned while placing the left hand in front of your heart. You can stay looking forward, or you can add a little twist and look up to the sky. Keep both hips down by touching the earth, and fill your body with sweetness.

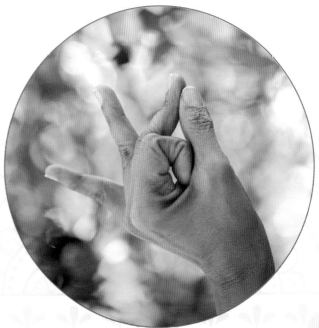

Pose 57

Ardha parighasana with *ardha pataka mudra*

Mudra

The mudras in song go like this: *pataka, tripataka, ardha pataka* . . . So here we come to learn another hand gesture called the half flag, or *ardha pataka*. We are going to use it here to show the bank of a river and then build our bridge upon it.

From *pataka*, flat palm, bend the ring and little fingers.

Asana

Come into kneeling position, pressing the knees and the tops of the feet down. Now open your right knee, bent at a 90-degree angle, to the right side, and place the right foot on the earth with the toes pointing to the right by your right hip. If you need to keep the hips down, move the right foot farther forward and ahead of the left knee. Now bring your hands to *ardha pataka*, place your right elbow on your right thigh, and lift your right hand to heart level. Lift your left arm up above your head, and side-bend deeper to the right. You can look forward or add a little bit of twist by shifting the gaze up to the sky.

This pose can be done in a more advanced variation with the right knee straight, the center of the right heel on the earth, and the right toes pointing up to the sky.

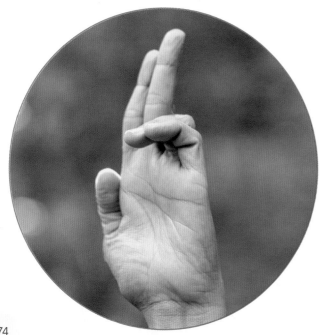

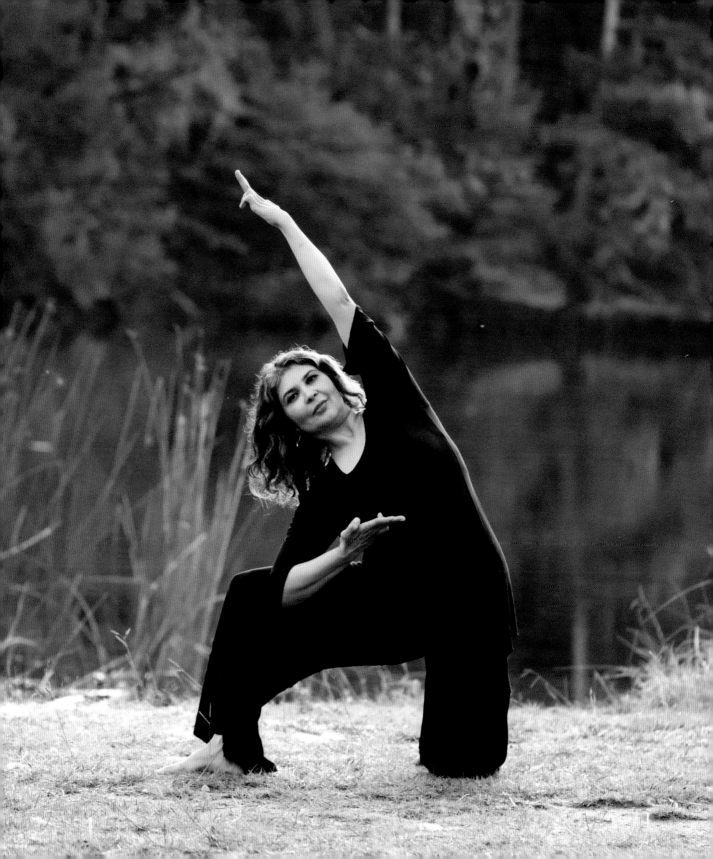

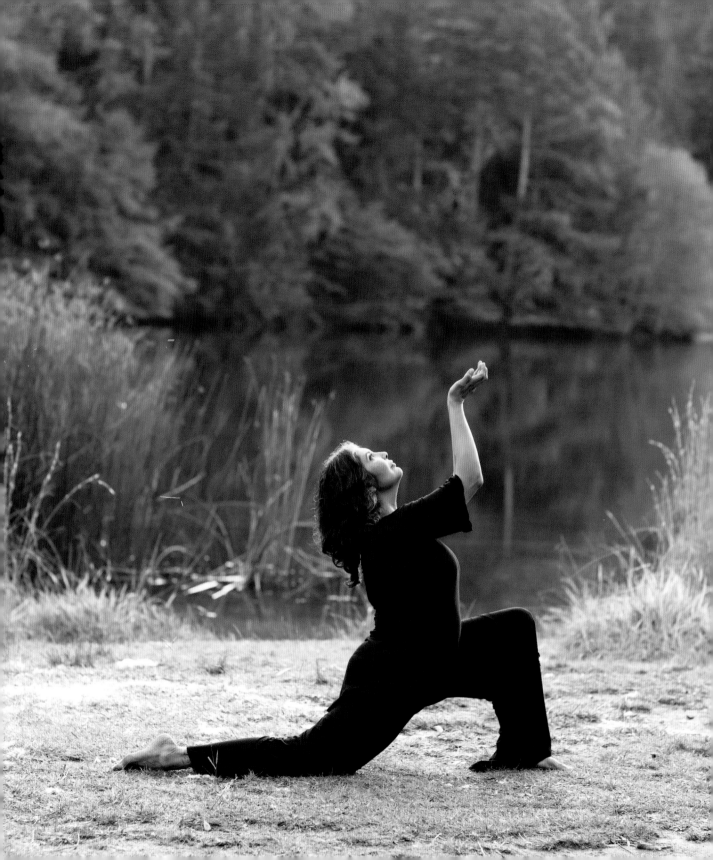

Pose 58

Anjaneyasana with *pushpaputa mudra*

Mudra

Pushpaputa is an offering mudra, and in this abhinaya it is a way of collecting water in your palms for washing your face, waking up with the blessing of the element of water and purifying your eyes and mind. It can be also a mudra of offering and receiving. As you hold it, imagine that you are inhaling and taking the light into your heart via your hands; as you exhale, you are offering the light of your heart to the world around you.

Bring your palms in *pataka*, flat with fingers together, and then bend your fingers slightly to make the shape of a bowl. Bring the little fingers and the outer edges of your hands to touch.

Asana

This pose is named after Hanuman as Anjaneya, the son of Anjani. Anjani was a beautiful *apsara*, or celestial dancer, who, because of her beauty, was cursed by an old sage who turned her face into a monkey face. Becoming a *vanara*, or one of the half-monkey, half-human race, she married Kesari and had Hanuman.

In this abhinaya, we are bringing a more feminine embellishment to Hanuman's asana and honoring Anjani's beauty.

Start by kneeling, and step your left foot forward to a 90-degree angle. Lower the hips to a low lunge while bringing the hands to *pushpaputa mudra* and slightly bending the back to open your heart to the sky.

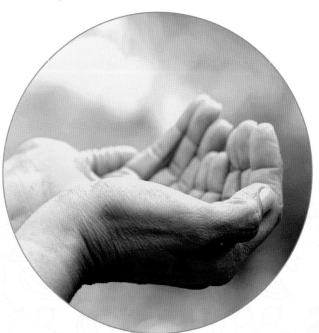

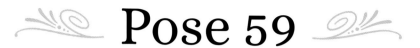

Pose 59

Anjaneyasana with *darpana* and *tripataka mudras*

Mudras

The *darpana mudra*, or mirror hand gesture, is engaged by simply flattening your palm to create a mirror at face level.

The *tripataka mudra* is used in this storytelling to show the placing of the kumkum, or red powder, as a bindi: a mark between and above the eyebrows as a sign of chastity and beauty.

This mudra and the mudra from the previous asana are used as part of a morning ritual to get ready for the day.

Asana

The low lunge can be done with the knee bent at a 90-degree angle, and you will feel the stretching happening more in the hip flexors. Alternatively, it can be done with a sharper angle, where the stretch will happen more in the Achilles tendon and calf. Depending on your joints, you can determine how deep toward the earth to move.

The backbend in this posture is optional; the important part is to connect with the mudra: If you are looking ahead, position your hand gesture at face level; if you are looking up, adjust your mirror.

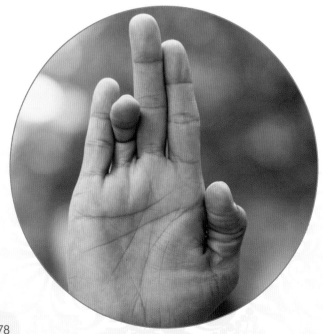

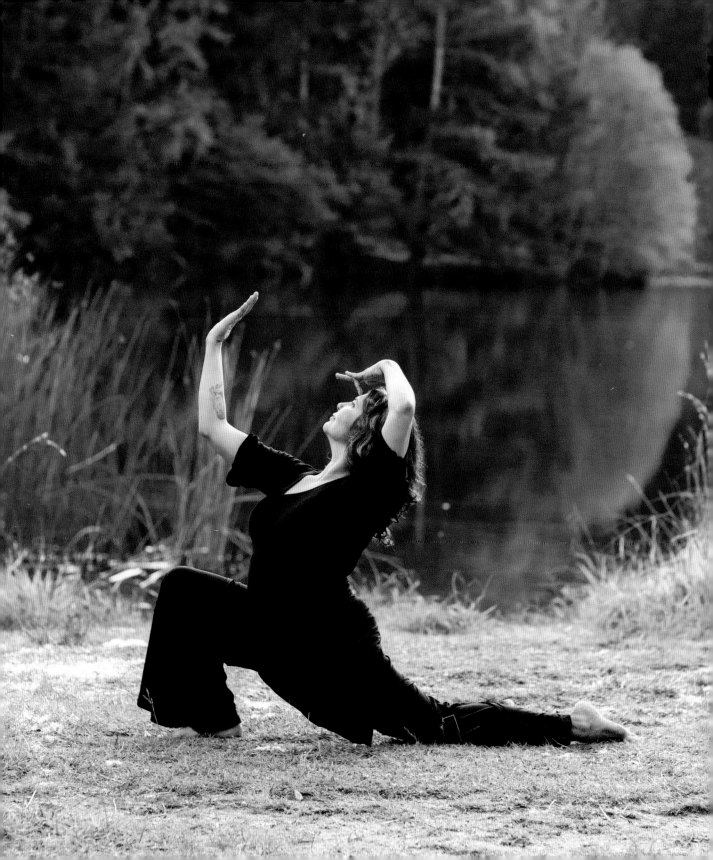

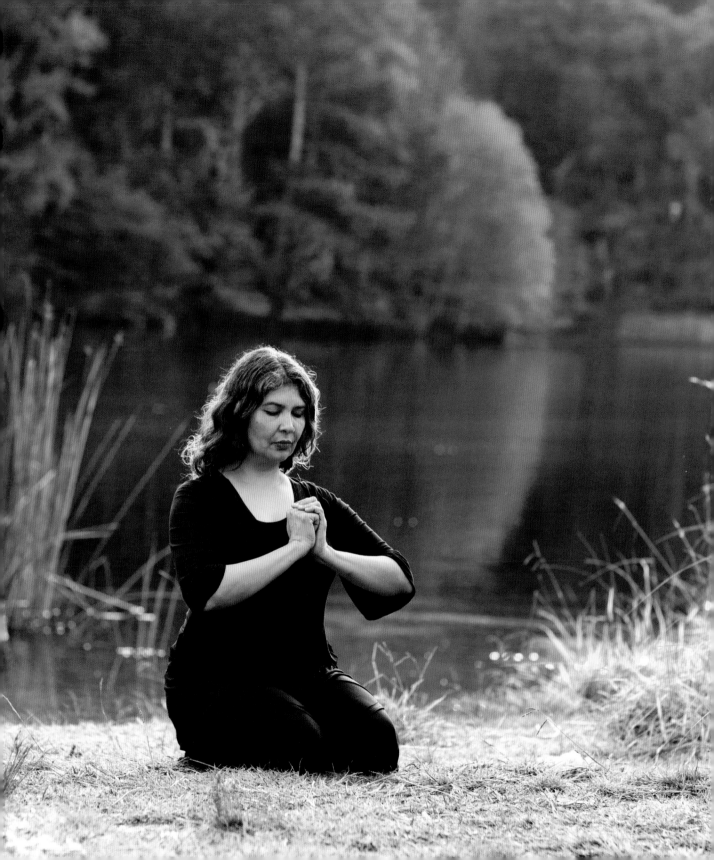

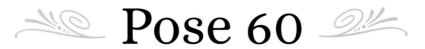

Pose 60

Vajrasana with *namrata mudra*

Mudra

Namrata means "humility," and this mudra shows it beautifully. This mudra is done in Odissi dance at moments of asking for forgiveness, though it is not an official Odissi mudra. I named it *namrata* and use it for meditation and to humbly ask for guidance. Close your right hand in a fist, *musti mudra*, and cover the fist with your left hand, bringing the hands in front of the heart and bowing your head slightly.

Asana

Vajrasana, or thunderbolt pose, supports the spine in an upright position for a while. It's a great pose for meditation. As you sit in this shape, you are blocking the flow of blood in the legs a little and increasing the flow of blood to the torso. In yoga, the torso is referred to as *kumbha*, or "the pot."

Simply sit on your heels with the knees and feet together. Focusing on your emotions and on the quality of devotion, sit in this pose and ask whomever you consider to be the highest for orientation.

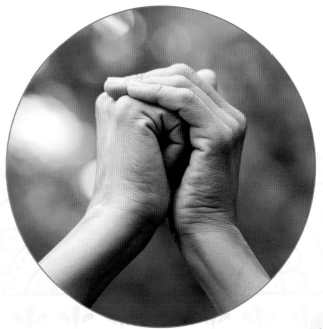

Pose 61

Ardha matsyendrasana with *Matsya mudra*

Mudra

Matsya, the fish avatar, comes to decorate this pose. Open your hands in *ardhachandra*, and from flat *pataka*, spread your thumbs out. Place one hand on top of the other such that the backs of your hands face up. This is another simple symbolic mudra that is filled with feeling and can be used in meditation to honor Matsyendranath and his hatha yoga legacy.

Asana

Sit on the ground and bend the knees to bring the soles of your feet to the ground while keeping the hips down. Keep your right knee up, and place your left knee under the right leg to bring the top of the left foot by the right hip and the left knee to the outer right foot. Embrace your right leg with your left arm, and place your right hand on the floor by your sacrum. Twist to the right as you shift your gaze back. Now bring your head to a neutral position while keeping the torso in a twist, bring your right hand to meet the left, and place the hands in *Matsya mudra* with the fingertips pointing down. You can shift your gaze over to the left shoulder.

This brings us back to Matsya as a little fish who watched Shiva teaching yoga to Parvati by the ocean while practicing it with devotion. In time, he evolves into the king of fish, Matsyendranath.

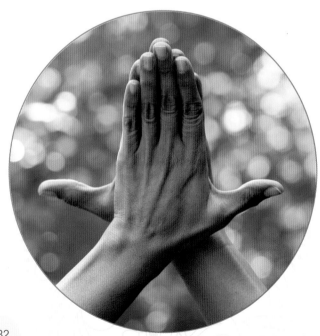

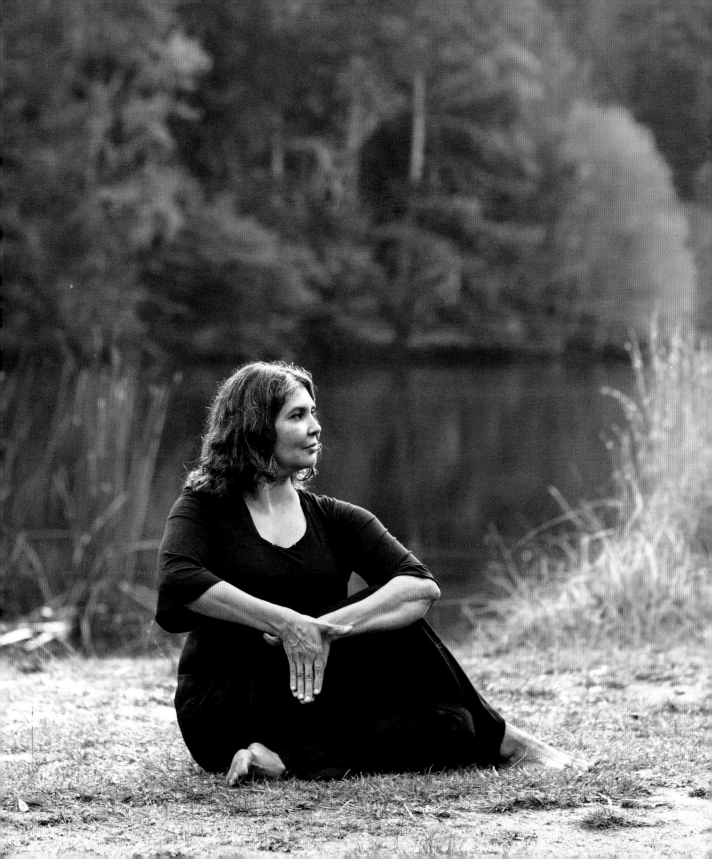

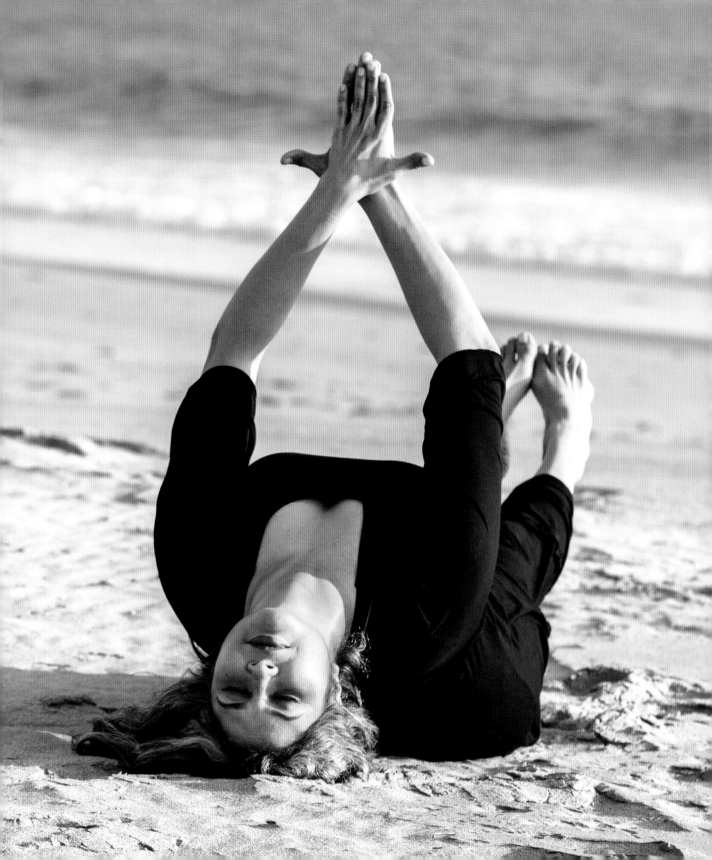

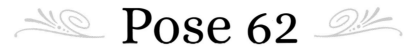

Pose 62

Matsyasana with *Matsya mudra*

Mudra

Matsya, the fish avatar, comes to decorate this pose. Open your hands in *ardhachandra*, and from flat *pataka* spread your thumbs out. Place one hand on top of the other so that the backs of your hands face up. This is another simple symbolic mudra that is filled with feeling and can be used in meditation to honor Matsyendranath and his hatha yoga legacy.

Asana

Lie on your back and bring your legs together, grounding them strongly on the floor while you point your feet. Lift your chest as high as you can to bring the crown of your head to the ground while arching the upper back into a backbend. Now lift your arms, place your hands in *Matsya mudra*, have your fish jump up from the envisioned water into the sky. If it feels right, elevate the legs for a more advanced variation.

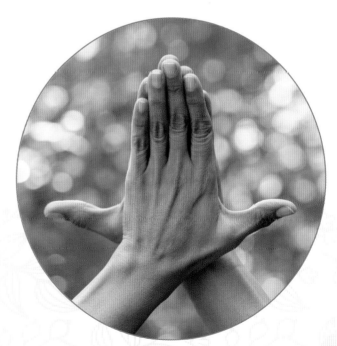

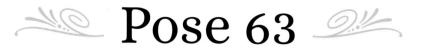

Pose 63

Garudasana with *Garuda mudra*

Mudra

For *ardhachandra*, form flat palms with thumbs open, and connect the pads of your thumbs while crossing your wrists and lifting your index fingers up toward the sky. Keep your fingers together.

Garuda is a mythical eagle deity, half eagle, half man, and he is the vehicle of Sri Vishnu. He is considered the protector of the dharma, as he attached himself to the preserver and serves as the preserver's vehicle, allowing Sri Vishnu's love and dharma to be distributed. Garuda's hands are often folded in *anjali*, or prayer mudra, showing his intention to serve.

Asana

I am showing a variation of the traditional *garudasana* that is much more accessible and more evocative to me personally. Begin by standing tall and opening your feet out. Bend your knees, and as you hold this shape, bring your hands to *Garuda mudra* in front of the heart center. Connect to the element of air within the heart, and ground deeply through your earthly feet. Now, transfer the weight to your left foot, and cross your right knee over your left knee while pointing your right foot up to the sky. Knee to knee is the key. Try to sit deeper on the left leg, and while lifting your right foot, add a little side bend to the left, and feel the right side stretching and creating this beautiful sculpture with your entire body.

Shape-shifting into your best self, carry on with your mission of supporting dharma and giving love.

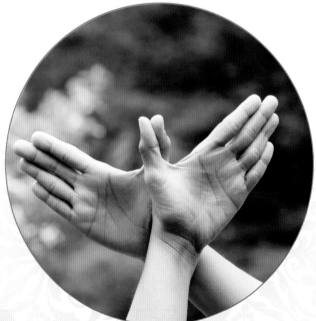

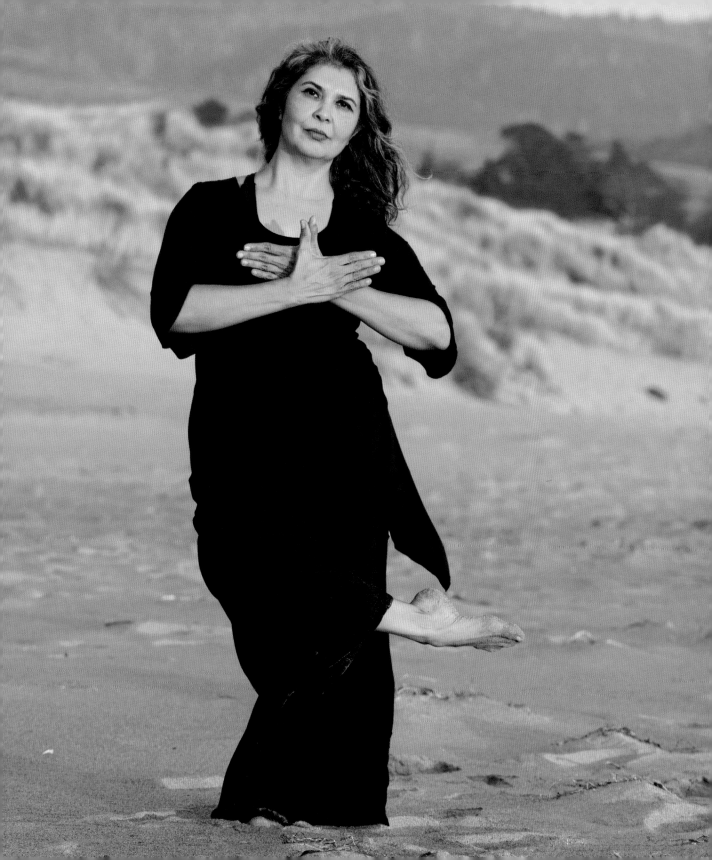

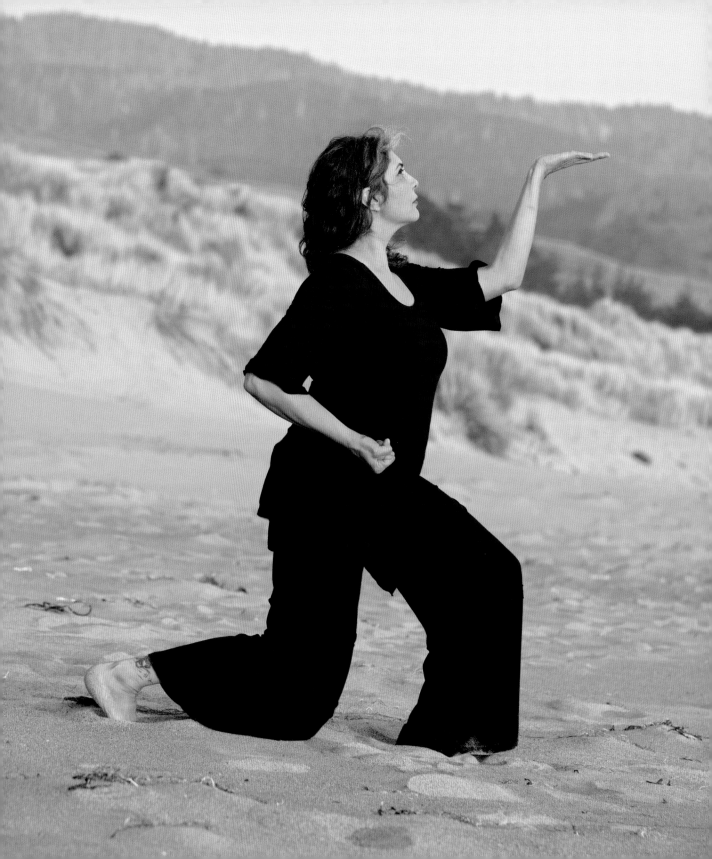

Pose 64

Hanuman sanjeevananagahatre bijasana with left hand in *pataka mudra* and right hand in *musti mudra*

Mudras

These two traditional dance *hastas* are combined here to tell the story of Hanuman flying through the sky while carrying Mount Dronagiri in his left hand, shown with *pataka mudra*, and carrying *bajarangi* or mace in his right hand, shown with *musti mudra*.

Hanuman's task was to find a healing herb called *sanjeevani* that would heal Lakshmana, who had been wounded on the battlefield. Not knowing which herb *sanjeevani* was, and not wanting to waste any time, Hanuman picked up the entire mountain and flew back to save Laskshaman.

Asana

Start in mountain pose, and step your right foot back about 2.5 feet. Bend your right knee as if you were going to touch the ground with your right kneecap, but don't. Bending your front leg, align your front knee over your front heel at a 90-degree angle.

In this Bhakti Nova pose, you are practicing to develop inner and outer strength. Your inner strength is one of resilience and service, and your outer strength is mainly of the lower body. There is a balance required in this pose, and as soon as you find it, add the mudras. Your left hand is in *pataka* with the palm up, and your right hand is in *musti*. Imagine that you are in the middle of an important mission, and let your dedication be completely focused on the completion of that mission. Although it is not scripturally traditional to hold the symbols on the other side, you can do it for the sake of balance, or you can simply stretch one arm up and one arm down.

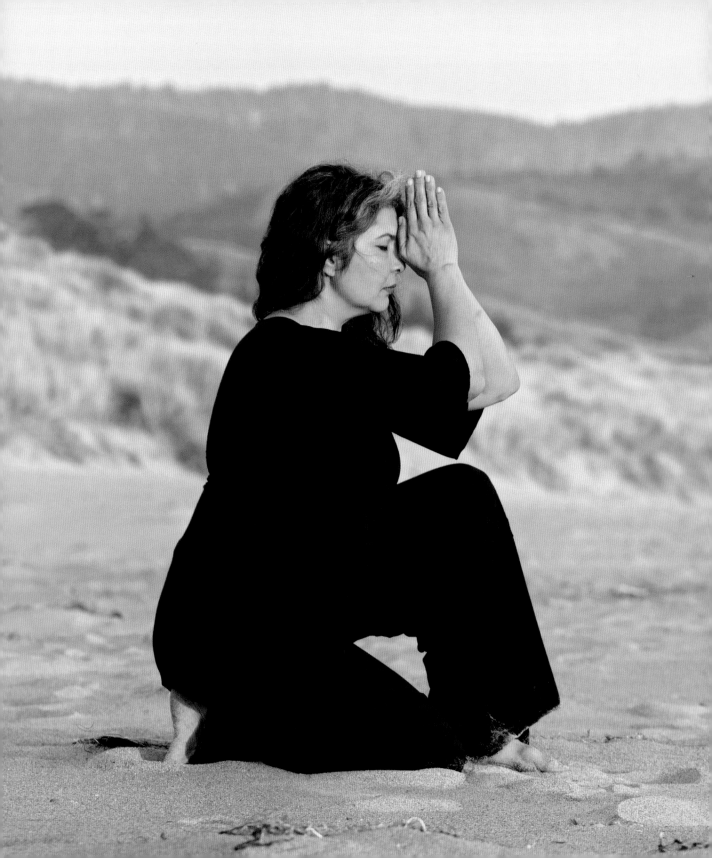

Pose 65

Hanuman bijasana, virasana variation with anjali mudra

Mudra

Anjali mudra is a hand gesture used for praying, and in this asana, it shows reverence and devotion. Hanuman is one of the most dedicated bhakta, and his example is to be followed.

Asana

Come into kneeling, and place the sole of your left foot by your right knee while sitting all the way back on your right heel. Lean forward, showing humility and respect, and bring your hands together in prayer to ask the one you serve: "How can I become an instrument of your light and love?" Asking for guidance, paying attention to the orders you receive, and executing those orders are the way of becoming a servant of God.

Sub Hari Bhaktan ki Jai!

All glory to the practitioners of devotion!

Closing Prayer
Blessings of light

· ·

*I pray that you may open your heart to receive
the blessings of light and love that are already
cascading down from the divine realm onto you. I
pray that you uncover your heart to be able to
see your own light shining within you and that this
light will be enough to bring you happiness and
satisfaction. Light all around you, and light within,
light guiding you, and light directing you back home.*

Om light om.

Om love om.

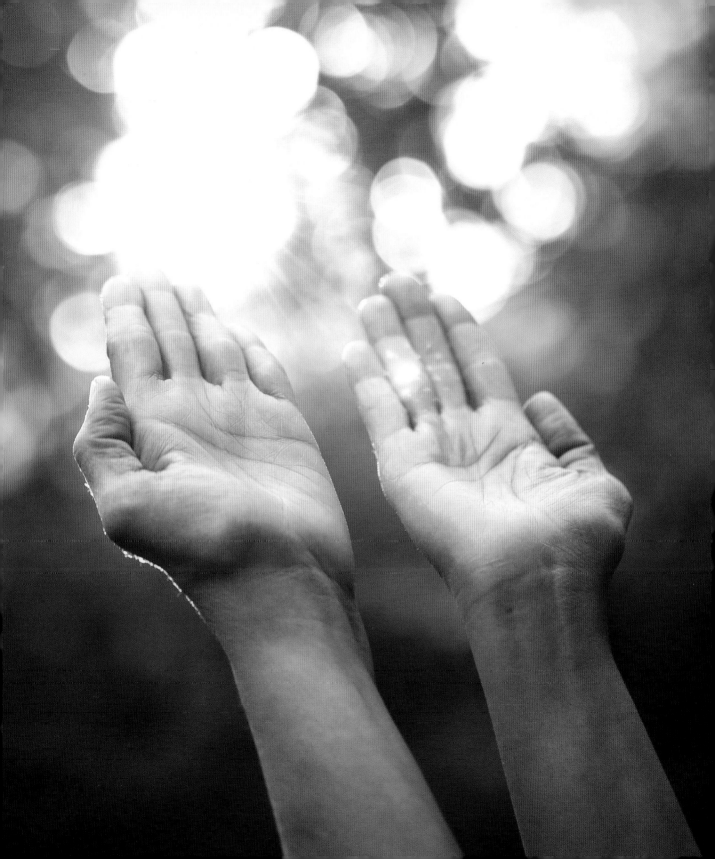

LIST OF ASANAS WITH MUDRAS

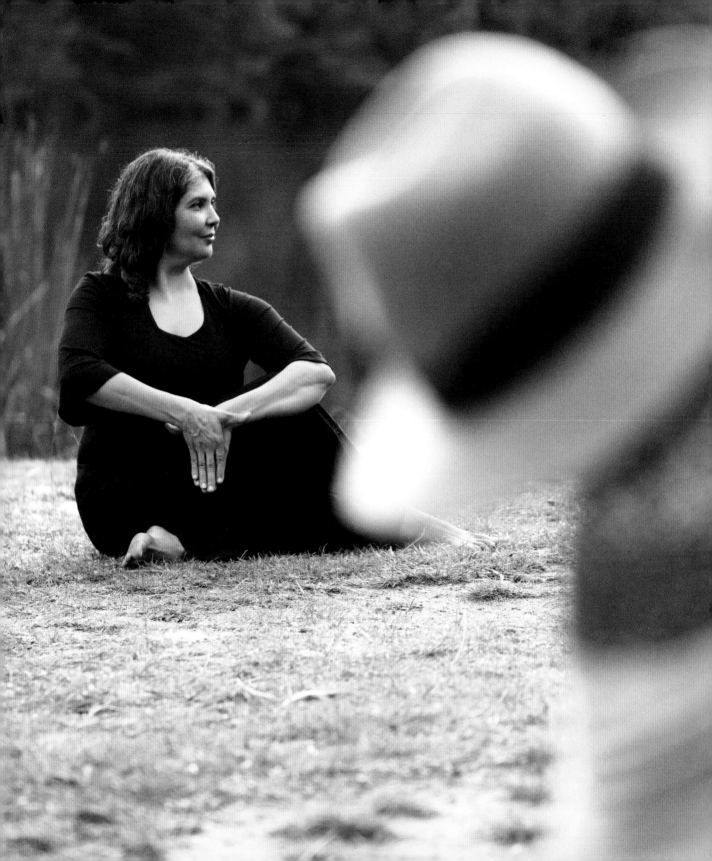

ACKNOWLEDGMENTS

I want to thank the universal mother, Jagadambe, for using her divine hands to make my human form. I want to thank my mother, Therezinha, for using her nurturing hands to hold me, love me, and shape me into an adult. I want to thank my father, Elias, for using his hardworking hands to provide for his children. I want to thank my extended family for using their constantly busy hands to direct, define, and guide me during my childhood.

I want to thank my first yoga teacher, DeRose, for using his knowledgeable hands to create a method of yoga that brought me into the hands of the ancient yoga. I want to thank Anderson Allegro, Shiva Rea, and all the yoga teachers that have supported me to grow on this path with their dedicated hands. I want to thank my first dance teacher, Sonia Galvão, for using her disciplined hands to mold the Odissi shapes in my body. I want to thank my dance guru, Vishnu Tattva Das, for using his devotional hands to infuse my Odissi shapes with Bhakti.

I want to thank Reiki master, Mikao Usui, and my Reiki teacher, Claudete França, for awakening in my hands the power of love through light. I want to thank my spiritual teacher, Lama Gangchen Rinpoche, for using his healing hands to rescue me and for giving me refuge in his unbroken lineage. I want to thank my spiritual mother, Siddhi Ma, who with her powerful loving hands showed me the deep meaning of service and love to the One. I want to thank the great orchestrator of my life, Neem Karoli Baba, for guiding me in this life and for waiting for me on the other side to hold my hands when this life is no more.

I want to thank my husband, Jai Uttal, who with his loving hands supports me in all of my creative and spiritual endeavors and inspires me with his daily devotion.

I want to thank my son, Ezra Gopal, who with his open hands and open heart teaches me how to receive and give love unconditionally. I want to thank my soul sisters—Lisa Maria, Kimberly Leo, Janice Gates, Naia Maro, Vasu, and many others—who with their Shakti-fied hands are constantly encouraging me to go forth on my path. I want to thank all of my students, who with their receptive hands allow me to pour what I have to give straight from my heart to theirs.

Specifically, for the making of this book, I want to thank my photographer and friend, Andrea Boston, who with her artistic hands helped me to manifest my dream into this beautiful offering. I want to thank my publisher, Raoul Goff, who with his intuitive hands answered my call and agreed so openly to the making of this book. I want to thank my editor, Pandita Geary, who with her precious hands received this project, saw it as a meaningful offering to you, and had to make miracles to correct my English. I want to thank my developmental editor, Linda Sparrowe, who, with her eagle eyes, saw the bigger picture of what needed to be birthed. Lastly, I want to thank the rest of the Mandala Publishing team (Phillip Jones, Amy DeGrote, Tessa Murphy, and so many more), who with their collective hands have created the right conditions for this book to be received by your hands right now.

Om Love Om

MANDALA

PUBLISHING

An Imprint of MandalaEarth

PO Box 3088

San Rafael, CA 94912

www.MandalaEarth.com

Find us on Facebook: www.facebook.com/MandalaEarth

Follow us on Twitter: @MandalaEarth

Library of Congress Cataloging-in-Publication Data available.

ISBN: 978-1-68383-644-5

Publisher: Raoul Goff

Associate Publisher: Phillip Jones

Creative Director: Chrissy Kwasnik

Designer: Amy DeGrote

Editor: Pandita Geary

Associate Managing Editor: Lauren LePera

Assistant Editor: Tessa Murphy

Senior Production Editor: Rachel Anderson

Production Manager: Sadie Crofts

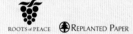

Mandala Publishing, in association with Roots of Peace, will plant two trees for each tree used in the
manufacturing of this book. Roots of Peace is an internationally renowned humanitarian organization
dedicated to eradicating land mines worldwide and converting war-torn lands into productive farms
and wildlife habitats. Roots of Peace will plant two million fruit and nut trees in Afghanistan and provide
farmers there with the skills and support necessary for sustainable land use.

Manufactured in China by Insight Editions

10 9 8 7 6 5 4 3 2 1